Education and
HIV/AIDS

Also available in the Education as a Humanitarian Response Series

Education and Reconciliation, Julia Paulson
Education as a Global Concern, Colin Brock
Education, Refugees and Asylum Seekers, Lala Demirdjian

Also available from Continuum

Children and Social Change, Dorothy Moss
Multiculturalism and Education, Richard Race
Sociology, Gender and Educational Aspirations, Carol Fuller

Education and HIV/AIDS

Education as a Humanitarian Response

Edited by

Nalini Asha Biggs

continuum

Continuum International Publishing Group

The Tower Building	80 Maiden Lane
11 York Road	Suite 704
London SE1 7NX	New York NY 10038

www.continuumbooks.com

British Library Cataloguing-in-Publication Data
A catalogue record for this book is available from the British Library.

ISBN: 978-1-4411-4778-3 (paperback)
       978-1-4411-6895-5 (hardcover)

Library of Congress Cataloging-in-Publication Data
Education and HIV/AIDS / edited by Nalini Asha Biggs.
     p. cm.
Includes index.
Summary: "Examines the relationship HIV/AIDS has with education in different international contexts, from Sub Saharan Africa, Southeast Asia, Eastern Europe, the USA, UK, and the Caribbean" – Provided by publisher.
ISBN 978-1-4411-6895-5 (hardback) – ISBN 978-1-4411-4778-3 (paperback)
1. HIV infections–Social aspects–Cross-cultural studies. 2. AIDS (Disease)–Social aspects–Cross-cultural studies. 3. Education–Health aspects–Cross-cultural studies. I. Biggs, Nalini Asha. II. Title.

RA643.8.E34 2012
362.196'97920071–dc22

                                                        2011016512

Typeset by Newgen Imaging Systems Pvt Ltd, Chennai, India
Printed and bound in India

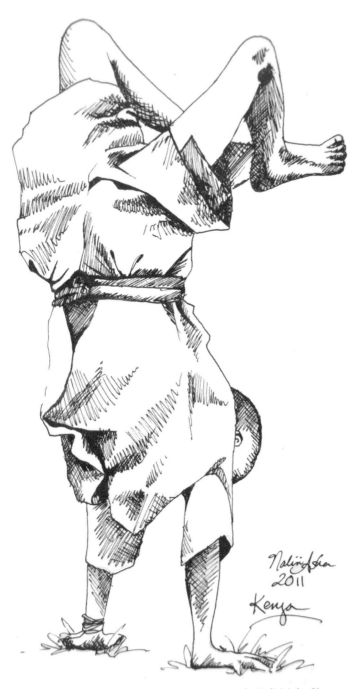

Deaf child doing a somersault across his schoolyard in Kenya, by Nalini Asha Biggs,
Pen and Ink, 2011

Contents

Series Editor's Preface

Underlying this entire series on *Education as a Humanitarian Response* is the well-known adage in education that "if we get it right for those most in need we will likely get it right for all if we take the same approach." That sentiment was born in relation to those with special educational needs within a full mainstream system of schooling. In relation to this series it is taken further to embrace the special educational needs of those experiencing disasters and their aftermath, whether natural or man-made. Much can be learned of value to the provision of normal mainstream systems from the holistic approach that necessarily follows in response to situations of human disaster such as a prevalence of HIV/AIDS. Sadly, very little of this potential value is actually perceived, and even less is embraced. Consequently, one of the aims of the series, both in the core volume *Education as a Global Concern* and the contributing volumes, such as this one, is to bring the notion of education as a humanitarian response to the mainstream, and to those seeking to serve it as teachers, educators in general, and politicians. The theme of *Education and HIV/AIDS* and the fact that this is one of the earliest of the volumes to be published is particularly apposite in that the range of countries experiencing HIV/AIDS spans the entire world. However, the most serious situations are found in low-income and middle-income countries in Africa, Asia, Latin America, and the tropical island zones, all of which exhibit a very wide range of contexts, problems, and responses. Such needs and the responses to those needs are well documented by the Inter-Agency Network for Education in Emergencies (INEE). Combating HIV/AIDS through various types of educational initiative should be in the forefront of radical thinking about the type of education we need to be fostering everywhere in order to be successful in the vital challenge of sustaining human and physical environments on planet Earth.

Colin Brock
UNESCO Chair in Education as
a Humanitarian Response, Oxford

Acknowledgments

I would like to thank Dr. Colin Brock for giving young academics like myself opportunities to share their ideas as well as Dr. Brock's friendship over the years. Thank you Dr. Mandisa Mbali for your insightful and detailed comments while drafting this book. I am grateful to my DPhil. supervisor, Dr David Mills, for being patient with this "slight" diversion, and to my colleagues and friends in the Department of Education and St. Antony's College for supporting me in so many ways. Thank you to the members of the Centre for Interdisciplinary AIDS Research at Oxford (CAIRO), for bringing to my attention many global and local issues that might otherwise be missed, and to Dr Lucie Cluver for organizing this group. Thank you to Jakki Odwesso for calling to my attention the significant and unusual circumstances of the Deaf community of Kenya in light of HIV/AIDS, and the Deaf women of Kibera and Dandora who shared with me the challenges they face daily. Thank you to my parents for supporting my goals, and to my dearest friend Heidi for *all the things!*

Most of all, I want to thank my wonderful husband and life partner, Travis, who learned to cook enchiladas the week the first draft of this book was due so that I wouldn't live solely off coffee and salami. Namaste.

Nalini Asha Biggs

Abbreviations and Terms

AIDS	Acquired immune deficiency syndrome
AIDS-related illness	Most commonly opportunistic infections such as tuberculosis and pneumonia, which kill because the immune system is impaired.
ART	Antiretroviral therapy
EFA	Education for All
FBO	Faith-based organization
HIV	Human immunodeficiency virus
HIV+	A positive diagnoses of the presence of HIV in the body
Incidence	With reference to HIV, the number of new infections per year per population, often a number projected from pregnant women who test HIV-positive at prenatal clinics.
Intervention	An action taken by an organization to reduce new infections, increase treatment or mitigate the negative impacts of this disease.
M&E	Monitoring and evaluation
MDG	Millennium Development Goals
MSM	Men who have sex with men
Malaria	Like a severe influenza, treatable and preventable, though often deadly with children or people with weakened immune systems such as PLWA, transmitted exclusively by mosquito bite
NGO	Nongovernmental organization
OVC	Orphans and vulnerable children
PEPFAR	The President's Emergency Plan for AIDS Relief, a US funding commitment
PLWH	Persons living with HIV
Prophylaxis	A measure taken to prevent a disease, such as a condom or ART, prescribed to reduce the risk of possible exposure to HIV infection

Prevalence	With reference to HIV, this is a percentage of people infected within a specific population, a number often projected from the numbers of pregnant women who test HIV-positive at prenatal clinics.
Serostatus	*Sero* refers to a virus; serostatus refers to the presence or absence of HIV in the body.
Serodiscordant Couple	A sexual paring in which one partner has HIV (whether he or she knows it or not) and the other partner is not infected
Sex Worker	A person who exchanges sex acts for goods, services or money
STI	Sexually transmitted infection
Stigma	A negative attitude towards a behavior, a social group, or an individual exhibiting a physical or mental difference, or idea; such an attitude is often realized through social exclusion or punishment. Stigma can be manifest, or feared as a potential manifestation. People react to manifest stigma and also to potential stigma.
Tuberculosis (TB)	Highly infectious, air-born illness (spread through coughing or saliva), which chiefly affects the lungs; previously called *consumption*, it is treatable with antibiotics and preventable with vaccine; it often kills young children or people with weakened immune systems such as PLWH.
UN	United Nations
UNAIDS	Joint United Nations Program on HIV/AIDS
UNESCO	United Nations Economic and Social Council
UNICEF	United Nations Children's Fund
USAID	United States Agency for International Development
VCT	Voluntary counseling and testing; often refers to the physical clinic where this happens
WHO	World Health Organization

Notes on Contributors

Jane Anderson is a consultant physician and Research Director at the Centre for the Study of Sexual Health and HIV at Homerton University Hospital NHS Foundation Trust in the United Kingdom. She holds honorary professorships at University College London and Queen Mary University of London, and is a member of the Executive for the Centre for the Study of Migration at Queen Mary University of London. She has clinical and research interests in HIV treatment and care, HIV in women and families, management of HIV in pregnancy, psychosocial aspects of HIV care and care of migrant and ethnic minority communities with HIV.

Nalini Asha Biggs is currently a DPhil. candidate in the Department of Education at the University of Oxford. She specializes in the sociology of HIV/AIDS and sex education for people with disabilities in developing countries, holding an MEd in International Education from the University of Sydney, Australia, and an MA in Special Education from San Diego State University, California. She completed her BA in Literature/Writing at the University of California, San Diego. Her current research focuses on schools for the Deaf in Kenya and as a classically trained artist she also illustrates her research fieldwork using a variety of mediums.

Christopher Castle is Chief of the Section of Education and HIV & AIDS in the Division of Education for Peace and Sustainable Development in UNESCO's Education Sector, as well as the UNESCO Focal Point for HIV and AIDS. With more than 20 years of experience working in education and development, he was also a research associate at the Horizons programme, led by the Population Council. Mr. Castle holds a BS in International Studies and French from The American University, Washington, DC and an MSc in International Relations from the London School of Economics.

David James Clarke is an independent consultant based in Bangkok, Thailand with a BSc in Sociology and a MA in Teaching English as a Foreign Language. He was formerly a senior education adviser with the Department for International Development in the United Kingdom, most recently with responsibility for the education response to HIV/AIDS and orphans and vulnerable children. He has more than ten years of experience in HIV-related work and has worked on policy, planning, programming, and evaluation in the education sector in sub-Saharan Africa, the Americas, and the Asia-Pacific region. He is the author of *Heroes and Villains: Teachers in the Education Response to HIV* (UNESCO IIEP, 2008).

Tuncay Ergene is an associate professor in the Counseling and Guidance Program at Hacettepe University in Ankara, Turkey, where he also has a degree in counseling. He holds MA and PhD degrees from Middle East Technical University in Ankara, Turkey, and Ohio University in Athens, Ohio, respectively. He completed postdoctoral studies in the International Mental Health and Developmental Disabilities Research and Training Program at Harvard University. Dr. Ergene is the president of the Turkish Psychological Counseling and Guidance Association and serves on the editorial boards of several journals.

David Kovara is currently an associate at the Middle East Office of McKinsey & Company, where he focuses on education reform in the Gulf Cooperation Council. Prior to McKinsey he was a Rhodes Scholar at the University of Oxford where he received a Diploma in Theology and a DPhil from the Department of Education. He also holds a BA in Philosophy from the University of Delaware. In 1998 he supported the foundation of the Children's Legal Action Network (CLAN) for abused children in Kenya, and has worked with local and international NGOs in both Nairobi and Kampala, including Doctors without Borders and the African Network for the Prevention and Protection against Child Abuse and Neglect (www.anppcan.org).

Priya Lall is currently a DPhil candidate in the Department of Social Policy and Social Intervention at the University of Oxford. She completed both her BA in Sociology and Politics and MA in Sociology at Warwick University in the United Kingdom. Her research interests are in gender, health, and social deprivation in developed and developing countries. She has previously researched mental coping strategies of Burmese refugees in a clinic on the Thai/Burmese border, social deprivation and unemployment in the United Kingdom, and social workers' experiences of catering to the needs of socio-economically deprived families.

Fadhila Mazanderani is a doctoral candidate at the Oxford Internet Institute of the University of Oxford, and a research associate at the University of Warwick Medical School in the United Kingdom. After completing an undergraduate degree in information technology (majoring in computer science and information systems) at the University of Pretoria, South Africa, she worked as a consultant specializing in media and telecommunications. Prior to starting her doctoral research on health-related internet use by people living with HIV, she completed an MA in New Media, Information and Society at the London School of Economics and Political Science.

Kerim Munir is Director of Psychiatry, Division of Developmental Medicine at the University Center of Excellence in Developmental Disabilities (UCEDD) and an associate in psychiatry in the Department of Psychiatry at the Children's Hospital, Harvard Medical School in Boston, Massachusetts. He is also the director of the Mental Health/Developmental Disabilities (MH/DD) Research Training Program at the Children's Hospital in Boston, which is funded by the Fogarty International Center and the National Institute of Mental Health in the United States of America. Dr Munir began international liaison activities between the United States of America and Turkey as a consultant to UNICEF in 1999, following two major earthquakes.

Mark Richmond is currently Director of the Division of Education for Peace and Sustainable Development in UNESCO's Education Sector as well as the UNESCO Global Coordinator for HIV & AIDS. He is responsible for education and HIV and AIDS, education for sustainable development, including the UN Decade of Education for Sustainable Development (DESD, 2005–14), and education for peace, human rights, and global citizenship. He graduated from the University of Sheffield in the United Kingdom with an honors degree in Political Theory and Institutions and has a MPhil in Comparative Education from the University of Hull in the United Kingdom.

Doreen Tembo is a Rhodes Scholar and social policy graduate of the University of Oxford's Department of Social Policy and Intervention. Her DPhil. thesis focused on social behavioral policies of HIV/AIDS prevention in resource-poor settings. She currently works as a research officer for the National Institute for Health Research and the University of Essex in the United Kingdom. Doreen has previously worked within the field of economic development, health policy, sexual and reproductive health, and demography with state, international aid, and technical assistance agencies and institutions of higher learning in Zambia and the United Kingdom.

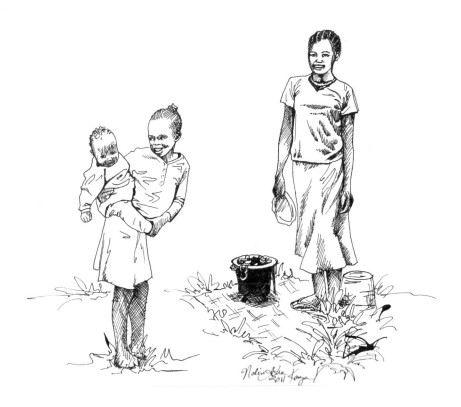

Two daughters of a head teacher cooking and looking after their younger brother, western Kenya, by Nalini Asha Biggs, Pen and Ink, 2011

Introduction

Nalini Asha Biggs

A young Kenyan mother sits on a wooden bench with her 6-month-old baby wrapped in a fuchsia and blue *kitenge* (traditional, African printed cloth) slung around her shoulders. Along with 40 other women she sits in this brightly painted room with wooden walls painted yellow and red and blue and green. The open wooden slats of the windows allow the cool breeze, mixed with the scents and smells of the Kibera slum. It's a hot, February afternoon in Nairobi.

She is here because a local NGO has paid her a small travel stipend so she can afford to spend three hours learning about birth-control methods, where to get tested for STIs and HIV, and how to use traditional medicines in case she needs to manage the symptoms of AIDS.

The young mother is lucky to have a few years of schooling though her literacy barely extends beyond managing to write her name on the sign-in sheet in order to claim her stipend of 250 Kenyan Shillings (about US$3). A handful of these women know they are HIV-positive and are encouraged by these meetings to manage their health through nutrition and knowing their human rights, while others are still unaware of their infection. Most of these women exchange sex for goods, services, or money on a regular basis, but do not identify themselves as sex workers. Instead, they have one or several "boyfriends" who pay for rent or food for their children. Some "service" the local police so that they are not arrested for begging in local bars. If they do sell sex—often for about the same price as a packet of condoms—they place a wooden stool outside the door of their corrugated shack to indicate that they are available for business.

For these Kenyan women, like so many others worldwide, HIV/AIDS is a daily threat. Still, they are afraid to get tested: they have no money to pay for treatment if they are HIV-positive and completing the paperwork to show they are too poor to pay is difficult when they only know a little written English or Kiswahili. Civil workers, in their experience, customarily demand bribes to ensure that the paperwork is not "lost." They have no surplus cash to pay for the *matatu* rides (small buses) across town. Still, the biggest fear compounding these technical challenges is potential stigma from being seen visiting a Voluntary Counseling and Testing (VCT) center. In the sprawling slums of Nairobi word travels fast, and they might be ostracized as "diseased," or worse, their children kicked out of their homes, and beaten by boyfriends or husbands for being "loose."

Besides, they tell the NGO workers after class, they are just as likely to die from malaria, TB, or some other infectious disease. Yes, HIV/AIDS is a serious threat and can kill you without treatment, but the possibility of death or disablement is a daily one.

The NGO worker tells them again how using condoms will not give them HIV and not all condoms "smell bad" as they mainly claim the government-provided ones do. They tell them that it is a myth that condoms can get stuck inside a woman and kill her, or that birth control pills make women infertile. She tells them safe sex can be "sweet sex," a slang term for sex good for both partners and a catch-phrase the NGO is trying to spread through the slums.

The women pay close attention, but bore quickly from this same old instruction, and side conversations spring up around the room. Then the facilitator asks for a volunteer to try and help the group understand today's theme through a personal story. Today the facilitator is trying to get the women to talk about *negotiation* with their male sexual partners so that they will have a better chance of discussing condom use, getting tested, and staying faithful to one person at a time. Hands shoot up around the room and as one woman is chosen, all eyes are fixated on her. She begins *signing* her story. These women are Deaf (see Biggs, 2010).

Like many who are very poor and with little education, these Deaf women have been treated all their lives as if their health doesn't matter. It is difficult for educators to fight both social exclusion and internalized myths of inferiority. These women are repeatedly surprised to hear they have the right not to be raped within marriage, and that they can't be turned away from medical care because they use sign language and writing to communicate. This vignette is replayed thousands and thousands of times around the world with other women, men, and children of varying abilities, disabilities, languages, cultures, religions, and races—all dealing with many injustices in their daily lives. Now on top of it all they must deal with HIV/AIDS.

What is education as a humanitarian response for these women? The rate of HIV infection in Kenya's population is around 8 percent. For the extremely poor, especially women who practice transactional sex, it is much higher. The layers of stigma these women live beneath have created a situation where they are more likely to become infected at a relatively young age with HIV, and less likely to know their serostatus, or obtain treatment. They and many like them worldwide have been denied an education; turned away from health clinics, legal, and social services; and often even from their own families and communities. To get by and to feed their children, they have often been forced into unequal and abusive relationships with men who are not sexually monogamous. They trade sex for money, food, housing, or protection and live in squalid "houses" made of scraps of steel, mud and plastic bags, with little to no sanitation or security.

Women with disabilities in developing countries represent a macabre case study of all the contextual factors, often stigma-related, that can exacerbate the risk of HIV infection and death from AIDS. This is the context they live within, and for education to be a humanitarian response, it must respond to these realities. More than just providing a few workplace skills like computer literacy or lace-making which indeed would provide them with some income and dignity, educators worldwide are increasingly recognizing the greater role education can play across multiple aspects of each human's life. Humanitarian education responds to the *entire* human.

What might such education look like in this context? For one, there are many points in these women's lives where simply being included in formal education might have "made the difference." Most people with disabilities worldwide are excluded from schooling or appropriate education. We can go even further and consider education as a humanitarian response for the people in their communities, namely those in power who currently limit their choices and freedoms.

Education as a humanitarian response views the Deaf women of Kibera not only as individuals, but also as part of a community, and of course as mothers. Many of the choices they make, though rather risky, are with their children in mind. They, like most parents, want something better for their children, and so will make sacrifices even of their own health and well-being to pay for school fees, medical care and other necessities. Making education costs less or none at all significantly opens up the choices these women have in life, especially over their sexual behavior.

"HIV/AIDS education" is increasingly defined not only by the transmission of information to encourage behavior change. It can mean talking to police, doctors, and lawyers about the human rights of each community's most vulnerable and stigmatized individuals. The "education response" to HIV/AIDS can be even more broadly defined, as encompassing education for social change to create a society where such a virus does not become an epidemic.

As I write this introduction, people around the world are celebrating World AIDS Day (annually on December 1) by wearing red ribbons and touting some of this year's slogans about a "prevention revolution." My *Twitter* feed and *Facebook* updates are full of advocacy messages for testing, reducing stigma, and increasing funding. Students and faculty have been gathering at my university to share their research and ideas for the future while in the media everyone from the U.S. President Obama to reality-television celebrities are making bold statements and promising action.

The HIV/AIDS "machine" is a monolithic thing: it has taken on its own culture and personality, impacting and interacting with virtually everything. Wearing the "red ribbon" is no longer limited to just public-health researchers, a few globally conscious celebrities, and the immediate families of people living with HIV. The "fight" has arguably saturated public discourse, though we have moved to calling it a "response" in order to lessen the stigma against those living with HIV.

Back in the early 1980s, most people first heard about HIV and AIDS through newspapers and television. While today we use our cell phones and the Internet to learn about new breakthroughs and updates, the basic activity remains the same: the transfer of information. We *learn* about HIV/AIDS but HIV/AIDS also impacts *how* and *what* we learn. Whether it's a private discussion with a nurse after getting our test results, taking a health class in high school, reading a billboard over a highway, or looking up AIDS on *Wikipedia*, we are educated by others as well as educating ourselves about this disease.

About this book

This book attempts to make explicit what so much research, policy, and practice make implicit: that in a world where HIV/AIDS impacts everyone's lives, education must in turn respond if it is to be humanitarian. This book also argues that there are as many different kinds of responses as there are contexts, and each epidemic requires local knowledge and action. Education must respond not only to the direct results of this disease, but the broader social, cultural, economic, and environmental contexts that make this epidemic possible and continue to feed it.

The authors of these chapters were specifically chosen because of their range of perspectives as well as significant specialization in a regional context. This book gives, therefore, a broad introduction into this subject while being supported by specific examples, either on a personal and local level, or by case study of a process or idea. In the "Global Overview," I first introduce the basics of HIV/AIDS medically and socially, both contexts to which humanitarian education responds.

Then we open with a chapter on the international response by Mark Richmond and Christopher Castle who both have extensive experience with UNESCO and who give an overview of which different agencies impact international policy as well as major documents that also have made changes along the way. David Kovara's chapter on a recent history of the President's Emergency Plan for AIDS Relief (PEPFAR) in the USA gives a rich account of the highly political nature of HIV/AIDS funding. Similarly, Doreen Tembo describes the politics of policy planning of the ABC strategy in Zambia. Priya Lall analyzes how the educational act of learning about their HIV status can reflect people's broader social and cultural contexts. David Clarke gives a policy overview of the educational response to HIV/AIDS in the Caribbean, highlighting its unique characteristics. Fadhila Mazinderani and Jane Anderson explore the evolving relationship between HIV/AIDS education and the Internet, with a case study of African immigrants in the United Kingdom. Finally, Tuncay Ergene and Kerim M. Munir describe the different ways HIV/AIDS and education interact in the unique context of Turkey.

Each of these chapters provides us with insight into the many different kinds of HIV/AIDS epidemics that have manifested worldwide as the greater pandemic, and how local context significantly changes the relationships between HIV/AIDS and education. They also give us lessons that can be generalized to similar contexts or serve as examples of what went wrong. Finally, each author also reminds us of the human side of this issue: that behind each statistic, policy, legal statute, and paper is a person, a family, and a community.

We encourage you to read critically and think to yourself how these ideas and lessons impact the way you think about education and HIV/AIDS and other similar health and social issues. These are only some of the myriad of perspectives that together make up what we know about this topic. The more perspectives there are from contexts that are unique or under-researched, the better we will be able to reduce infections and increase the standard of living of those who are HIV-positive while at the same time shaping education to be increasingly a truly humanitarian response.

Reference list

Biggs, N. A. (2010). "Adapting HIV/AIDS Education for Deaf Kenyans and the Impact of Local Context." Presentation at the XVIII International AIDS Conference, Vienna, Austria (July 23).

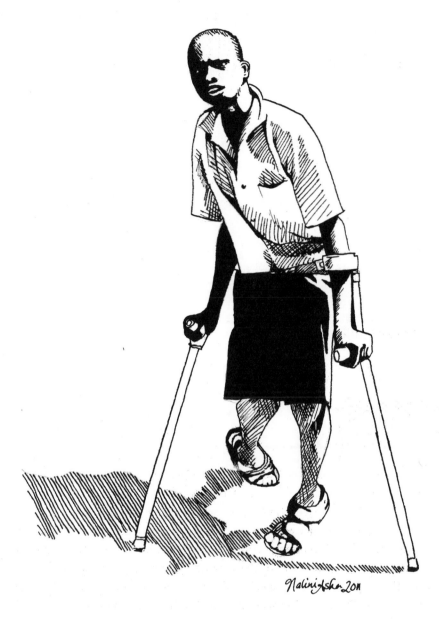

A young man with multiple disabilities in a school for the Deaf, western Kenya, by Nalini Asha Biggs, Pen and Ink, 2011

Global Overview

Nalini Asha Biggs

What is HIV/AIDS, and why does education matter?

The purpose of this global overview is to provide a succinct but accurate background based on the most recent research as of early 2011 for nonspecialist readers interested HIV/AIDS and education. The following chapters provide more in-depth examinations of specific regional issues and political, social, cultural, and economic contexts that make for very different epidemics worldwide. For more thorough data and discussion, please follow the citations that have been chosen specifically for the purpose of further reading on these issues. The following section provides the reader with a basic knowledge of the medical and social aspects of this disease to which "humanitarian education" must respond.

Terminology

Initially in the early 1980s public health officials at the Centers for Disease Control in Atlanta in the United States of America identified an epidemic of a new, infectious, and fatal disease that seemed to kill off a person's immune system. This collection of symptoms was soon called the acquired immune deficiency syndrome, or AIDS. It was later discovered that a virus causes this condition. The human immunodeficiency virus, or HIV, enters the blood stream, injects its genetic code into the very white blood cells (CD4 immune cells) needed to fight off such diseases, remains dormant for years, and then emerges to destroy the infected person's immune system.

AIDS therefore describes the physical state, or more specifically, set of conditions, where consequently a person's immune system is so depleted that he or she becomes extremely vulnerable to opportunistic infections. HIV-positive individuals then begin to show symptoms of the kinds of diseases that are associated with the syndrome such tuberculosis, one of the biggest killers. Taking medication can significantly slow the progression of HIV, allowing for significant immune-system recovery. People may come into a hospital severely weakened, extremely thin (in some parts of the world, the colloquial term for AIDS is *slim*) and thinking they will die. Once they begin antiretroviral therapy (ART), they gain weight, feel stronger, and are able to return to a somewhat normal life. ART therapy is now recommended by WHO for all people living with HIV with a CD4 cell count of below 350 and who have active TB (WHO, 2009). Such combination antiretroviral therapy requires over 95 percent adherence to be optimally effective. However, the majority of the people in the world who have reached this point do not get treatment and they will suffer greatly, and die fairly rapidly.

Although people commonly refer to "dying from AIDS," it is more accurate to say that death comes from an AIDS-related illness or illnesses. This is because people living with HIV who cannot access treatment actually die from one of the many common infectious diseases that are normally present in their communities that without HIV would probably be curable, or their symptoms even barely noticeable.

HIV, the virus that causes AIDS, is passed from individual to individual and reprograms antibodies to reproduce themselves. When there are so many copies of the virus (HIV) that the immune system is overwhelmed and ineffective, the condition is referred to as AIDS.

For the purposes of this book, in general, HIV and AIDS will usually be referred to together as HIV/AIDS. The "education response" often tries to reduce HIV transmission as well as prevent progression to AIDS through both timely initiation of treatment and adequate adherence. The stigmatizing, invisible HIV infection as well as the disability and death caused by AIDS *both* impact education. Education impacts *both* new infections, the progression to AIDS and subsequent death. We will at times refer to HIV and AIDS separately, but only when appropriate, such as "HIV infection" or "AIDS-related deaths."

Especially in terms of "prevention education," it is important to note that any education about either HIV or AIDS, including education on treatments, is always a kind of prevention. It is true that we largely hope to eradicate new HIV infections entirely, but in delivering the information people need to ensure regular testing and adherence to treatment, we are in fact also preventing AIDS and AIDS-related deaths. In educating people about HIV treatments that lower the probability of transmission of the virus, we are also helping to prevent further spread as people who are aware of their status receive regular counseling and those who are on ARTs are less likely to infect others with whom they come into contact (Cornman et al., 2008; Gilbert et al., 2008).

In terms of stigma especially, HIV and AIDS are difficult to separate. Stigma is a recurring theme in this book and central to understanding the relationship between HIV/AIDS and education. It is largely through education that we can reduce stigma on many levels. As with the story of the Kenyan Deaf women, there are issues of stigma surrounding the testing process and of the moral assumptions of their community, all of which make HIV/AIDS more reliant on the local and even distal attitudes and beliefs about sexuality and morality than other illnesses. Several contributing authors in this book analyze the ways that stigma has impacted how people seek or receive education on HIV/AIDS, as well as how education can lessen or transform stigma. In each instance, the line between HIV and AIDS is almost nonexistent or unimportant. For these reasons we use the term *HIV/AIDS*; you will see that we only rarely make reference to HIV and AIDS separately.

Why is this an epidemic?

How HIV is transmitted is also of the upmost importance for understanding its relationship with education. With only rare exceptions, people become infected in the most intimate of social situations: during the exchange of certain bodily fluids during sexual intercourse or sharing needles during drug use. The large majority of new infections each year, around 2.7 million in 2007 alone, is increasingly through heterosexual intercourse, especially in sub-Saharan Africa, but to a lesser extent elsewhere (Dosekun and Fox, 2010; UNAIDS, 2008). Not all fluids infect equally, and not all sexual acts involve the same risk of transmission. HIV is passed most efficiently through blood and semen, through breast milk, and to a much lesser extent through vaginal secretions. For this reason a good deal of discussion in this book centers on sexual activity, though the other common transmission pathways are referenced when appropriate.

Sexual transmission

Men and women who are receiving anal sex without a condom are most at risk of contracting HIV with the average risk being between 0.04 and 3.0 percent *per sex act* (when the penetrative partner is HIV-positive and the receptive partner is HIV-). Women engaging in vaginal sex without a condom are the next most vulnerable group, which is right now the fastest growing pathway to infection worldwide, especially in sub-Saharan Africa (Fox and Fidler, 2010). The anal cavity is especially susceptible to cuts that allow for the direct transmission of HIV from seminal fluids to the blood stream because it is delicate and not naturally lubricated. The vaginal canal, while ideally well-lubricated, is also easily torn, and even the smallest of cuts makes a perfect pathway for HIV to enter the bloodstream. For women, forced sex, which can often mean abrasions and cuts to the genitalia, can increase their risk of infection. "Dry sex" is also sometimes preferred in some cultures, especially in Africa, and women will intentionally dry out the natural fluids before having sex. Adequate lubrication, for either anal or vaginal penetration, also reduces the chances of tears in the condom.

Whether a man is circumcised or not also impacts the chances of transmission, reducing it by 60 percent in some efficacy trials studies (Auvert et al., 2005; Baily et al., 2007; Gray et al., 2007), though it only protects the penetrative partner who already has a lower risk per act when the receptive partner is HIV-positive. Re-trials of some studies have later showed lower efficacy (between 51–53%), and these controlled studies only represent a potential rarely found in the real world. These studies also only address female to male transmission; a circumcised man is possibly protected against infection by others but can just as easily pass on HIV to his partners. These studies give little hope to the women of the world who are increasingly at greater risk of infection.

Having other STIs, especially those that are untreated, makes this even more dangerous, as the very immune cells that are attracted to the open sores of STI-related inflammation are what HIV must attach to in order to infect an individual. This is why education about preventing new infections necessarily requires talking about all kinds of common STIs, and ways of reducing small cuts and tears in the anal cavity and vaginal wall, which allow for extremely easy infection.

Sharing needles for drug use

Sharing needles is by far the quickest way to become infected as the immediate transfusion of even trace amounts of HIV-infected blood into one's own blood stream is an extremely efficient means of transmission. Because of the ease of transmission through the exchange of blood through sharing needles, drug users *ought* to be the most targeted population for prevention. However, in contexts where HIV rates are high even among the general population and not pocketed within "higher risk groups," educational campaigns often attempt to reach many groups of people all with the same kind of education. In these contexts, resources are scarce and the stigma attached to "risk groups" is already high, and so targeting education on such groups can be at times counterproductive. It is also difficult to secure separate funding and support for stigmatized risk groups.

Almost as a rule, the major barriers to this kind of education have little to do with the availability of scientific evidence or medical or educational resources. The research findings on what is needed to reduce HIV infection among this population are very clear, and this case is a perfect example of how law, public opinion, and political action can vary immensely and even contradict scientific evidence.

Mother to child

Without adequate treatment approximately one in three pregnant women who are HIV-positive will pass on the infection to their child in utero, during childbirth, or most commonly through breastfeeding. Where *vertical transmission*, or mother-to-child transmission (MTCT), is more common, especially in eastern and southern Africa, education is vital in combating cultural tradition and stigma regarding the substitution of breastfeeding with formula feeding when a mother is likely to otherwise infect her child. Using formula, though rather common and seemingly innocuous from a Western point of view, can be stigmatizing and economically crippling for many mothers, especially in rural Africa. It can be stigmatizing if a woman does not breast-feed her child in a culture where this is not only the norm, but one of the major ways a mother is expected to care for her child and symbolic of womanhood and integral to religious and cultural beliefs about nurturing. If a woman fails to breast-feed, she often fears that others will assume she is unfit, does not care for her child or is "cold." Drug treatments are now available to significantly reduce risk through breast-feeding, but they also require the provision of education to convince mothers to begin and adhere to treatment (Burke, 2004).

Other transmission pathways

Fortunately, blood supplies through concerted efforts, are an extremely minor route of infection and the number of clinical/hospital accidental needle-stick injuries or other clinical errors has been significantly reduced, especially in high-income countries. It is yet unclear to what extent the act of female or male circumcision might be spreading HIV, though it is certainly possible as such procedures are often conducted in unsterile conditions.

While there are theoretically many ways to become infected with HIV, they are either unlikely enough that education will help or are accidents in what is otherwise a controlled environment, such as a hospital where simple precautions and rules have virtually erased the risk. We have also reduced such accidents by simply increasing the overall awareness of blood-related infectious diseases and raising health facilities' hygiene standards.

The viral timeline

Compounding the problem of these risky sexual behaviors and other infection pathways is the viral timeline of HIV in the bodies of the estimated 33 million HIV-positive individuals. At about six weeks after infection, the infected individual's viral load reaches to an extremely high count, which is not matched until around seven to nine years later when AIDS begins to allow opportunistic diseases to weaken and finally kill the individual (Pantaleo, 1993). Meanwhile, during those first few weeks, the individual has no physical indication of his or her infection and often continues with the same sexual behaviors that produced the infection in the first place, spreading the virus to other partners. A study of *serodiscordant* (one partner is infected, the other is not) heterosexual couples in Uganda showed that the risk of viral spread per sexual intercourse during those first 2.5 months when one partner was infected was *twelvefold higher* than during later months and years (Wawer et al., 2005).

This is why regular HIV testing and consistent condom use is so vital, as well as getting treatment and adhering to it as soon as HIV has been diagnosed (Vernazza et al., 2008). In the United States of America alone, *half* of all infections are transmitted by people who *are not aware of their status* (Marks et al., 2006). In Africa, this jumps to 80 percent (WHO, 2008). Antiretroviral therapy, or ART, reduces the viral load to postpone the onset of AIDS as well as reduce the risk of infection to others, with some research showing a 95 percent reduction in transmission (Donnell et al., 2010).

These "vulnerabilities" and physical characteristics of HIV are best understood, however, in the socio-cultural context of transmission. The way we discuss this epidemic can have a real impact on the lives of people affected. Paula Treichler presents critical perspectives on the social constructions of AIDS research in her book *How to Have Theory in an Epidemic: Cultural Chronicles of AIDS* (2002). For instance, scientists may find a statistical difference between the risk factors of two kinds of sexual behavior, such as vaginal versus anal, but the cultural and political climate this science is embedded within can exaggerate these differences, stigmatizing individuals and groups. The language of HIV/AIDS is ever-changing as both advocates and researchers (often with dual-identities), recognize the impact terminology and discourse have on individuals. "People living with HIV" or PLWH has replaced "patient" or "victim." "Safe sex" to be rephrased as "safer sex," as no sexual act truly without risk, and many married people especially feel that they are not at risk of infection. See the 2008 UNAIDS publication on *Terminology Guidelines*, (available online at www.UNAIDS.org), for more discussion on the changing language of HIV/AIDS.

What are the limits of education?

Because of these characteristics, HIV/AIDS education often means sex education, and education on the other behaviors leading to higher-risk sex, such as drug and alcohol use, human rights and self-esteem, and reproductive health. Using drugs and alcohol significantly impacts the extent to which people engage in risky sexual behavior, and educating people on these topics can impact the contextual factors that lead to reducing HIV transmission (Yankah et al., 2008). These interventions are what most people think of when they hear "HIV/AIDS education," and tend to use *individual behavior change* strategies which are based on sociocognitive theories that argue that if people have the necessary facts, they will make better, more informed decisions (see Rosenstock, 1974). The efficacy of this kind of education directly relates to the range of choices and freedoms available to individuals to make those informed decisions. Educating people about the facts of HIV/AIDS can be only truly humanitarian when offered in a context that supports human rights, or alongside efforts to increase those rights.

Many argue that the local and individual situations in which HIV transmission is present involve very little rational decision making based on the facts of HIV/AIDS alone. Instead, decisions are made under the pressures of cultural, social, and sometimes biological factors that significantly limit choices.

For instance, think back to the women from the Kenyan anecdote. Even after they seek out and obtain adequate knowledge of HIV transmission, testing, and treatment, they still ask, "How do I turn away my boyfriend for sex? Who will feed my children?" Or, "If I go to the VCT, they see that I am Deaf, that I use sign language, so they turn me away" (Biggs, 2010). One of the more obvious cases illustrating lack of choice to make rational decisions is found in prison populations where forced sex or reusing shared needles is common. Another group is the married women in regions and communities where women's rights within marriage are minimal, making the discussion of condoms, getting tested, or seeking treatment virtually impossible. These are some of the major limitations to HIV/AIDS education, especially when viewed, as it sometimes is, as a "vaccine." Thinking of education, especially *individual behavior change* education, as a "magic bullet" can be dangerous without the complement of the technologies (free or low-cost condoms, testing services, ARTs) and community-wide respect for human rights, which are required for true choice in potentially infectious situations (UNAIDS, 2009).

HIV/AIDS-related technologies and education

Microbicides

The latest developments in "technologies" to prevent spread of HIV include variations on the use of ARTs as a prophylaxis, in the form of vaginal and anal microbiocide gels, or even in pill form (Veronese et al., 2010). Gels come in a packet, similar to that of a single-use lubricant, and are applied to the inside of the vagina or rectum as much as several hours before sexual intercourse. Education about this new technology might not change much from education about other methods in which nurses, teachers, and social workers would simply discuss the benefits of these gels or pills and how to negotiate using them with unwilling partners. Yet despite the significant gender inequality in most of the relationships where infection occurs, the development of a female-controlled and somewhat invisible prevention method is something to give us hope.

Condoms

There are many issues surrounding condoms. Because of the common taboos surrounding condoms as well as prevalent resistance to using them by both men and women, many hope that the development of a prophylaxis for women to use without others' knowledge will impact the spread of HIV. Research has found that across cultures and socioeconomic status, men are very resistant to using condoms, even when they are well versed in the benefits. Men often feel that using condoms reduces the pleasure of sex but also in many cultures the act of ejaculating into a woman is tied to manhood and health, and to prevent this act carries significant negative connotations. Condoms are also frequently viewed as a Western tool and are suspected of *causing* HIV/AIDS or a greater risk of infertility or miscarriage. Across many cultures there are sayings and phrases that reflect negative attitudes towards condoms. Some men compare using a condom to "eating candy with the wrapper still on" (see Basuki et al., 2002; Volk and Koopman, 2001; Yotebieng et al., 2009). These aesthetic reasons for not using condoms are also reported when female condoms are introduced (Thompson et al., 2006).

This does not even touch the issue of moral beliefs tied to condoms, often based on specific religious doctrine. While there is no research to support such beliefs, many still argue that the promotion of condoms as a prevention tool encourages young people to have sex. Many Catholics, as well, believe that any kind of contraception is religiously unacceptable, and only in 2010 did the pope finally admit that the use of condoms in the case of transactional sex between men in order to prevent HIV was acceptable. For sub-Saharan Africa, especially, where the influence of Christian churches is significant, this news was of special interest, though it is yet unclear to what extent this will change attitudes. David Kovara, in his chapter on PEPFAR, discusses how Christian, right-wing lobbies and interest groups in the United States of America made a significant impact on international funding policy, especially in terms of condom promotion, successfully reserving a third of all prevention funding for abstinence-only education. Doreen Tembo also discusses this issue in Zambia with similar results. "Abstinence education" can range from simply promoting abstinence and being faithful in marriage as a best-case scenario to be encouraged to outright defamation of condoms and other forms of contraception by educating people only on their limitations, with no mention of benefits.

In spite of these challenges, one of the main successes we have seen is increased use of condoms worldwide, and especially in sub-Saharan Africa where intense marketing campaigns have focused on the real benefits of condoms. While we wait for a vaccine, better and cheaper treatment and societal changes to decrease HIV incidence, condoms are still arguably the best hope we have for saving lives.

Antiretroviral therapy (ART)

As a self-described AIDS researcher I am often asked the rhetorical question, "Is AIDS *really* still a problem when we have drugs for that now?" While it is true that there is treatment available that make HIV a manageable chronic illness and these have saved the lives of many, these are unfortunately a lucky few. Most people who have HIV do not live in circumstances that make it possible to take advantage of these medicines.

For instance in many parts of sub-Saharan Africa where the epidemic is at its worst there is only enough medicine to treat a *third* of the number of people who need to begin therapy or likely soon die. These are individuals who have been infected for years and are at a significant stage of HIV and does not include the recently infected, a much larger population. Even if these medicines are provided at low or no cost and the individuals who need it can physically reach the dispensary and maintain the regimen, there is not enough to go around. This is the unfortunate reality of the current state of treatment.

Geography, adverse and extreme weather, cultural stigma and fear, political unrest, tensions with donor countries and economic insecurity or crisis all culminate in the areas where HIV is most prevalent. These factors all make adherence to scarce treatment difficult at best. While scientists work diligently to develop a vaccine that will fight against the most common strains of HIV, most countries are looking to education (whether in school or a broader definition) in order to prevent new HIV infections.

Who should be targeted for HIV/AIDS education?

We described first the kinds of behaviors that have shown to have a higher risk of infection, rather than focus on "risk groups" or people commonly associated with these behaviors. For educational responses and education in light of this epidemic, however, grouping people together by common behaviors can be useful in targeting scarce resources or focusing specific messages where they are needed most. They can also backfire, which we will return to later in section, by increasing the stigma of associating "riskier" behaviors and HIV/AIDS with entire populations.

In the conversations leading up to the writing of this book, Priya Lall, one of the volume's authors, once made explicit the kind of obvious yet poignant observation that so much research has made implicit: "It's not how risky your behaviors are, it's your choice of partners." That is to say, while most sexually active people engage in what we here would call "riskier" sexual behaviors the risk itself is also largely derived from "who" the partner of choice is (see Kenyon et al, 2009; Macintye et al., 2001). This is especially true when there is little choice for one of the partners or when one or both partners have little choices in life. "Higher risk" sexual behavior describes both physical vulnerability and a social context in which the act takes place.

Men who have sex with men, and gay men

Gay men are often targeted for campaigns on safer sex practices and to be tested for STIs and HIV; at the very start of the epidemic the Gay community in the USA was instrumental in advocating the need for such education, significantly influencing research and policy through their leadership in the AIDS response even before scientists fully understood the disease.

Educational campaigns specifically targeting gay men seems to have helped, as incidence in the USA, for example, has until recently declined. In countries and communities where it is difficult or impossible to be openly gay (because of laws and extreme social stigma), such education may prove ineffectual. In these contexts, increasing human rights and lessening the stigma of different sexualities and sexual practices might be more helpful. Because of this issue, AIDS research discusses sexual behavior more often than identity (where appropriate), and using the phrase "men who have sex with men" (MSM).

When homosexuality is not acknowledged or severely persecuted in a community, targeted educational campaigns can actually increase violence and stigma against those who are suspected of being gay, or who are attempting to secure their rights, by strengthening the notion that this group is "diseased," and "immoral." Fear of increased stigma can drive men to engage in riskier sexual practices such as sex work. Educational efforts have the challenge of balancing recognition of local cultural realities and potential ideals.

People who identify as having a sexuality or gender not commonly accepted by local cultures or political structures face not only social stigma but often unintentional invisibility within research practices. For instance Elizabeth Pisani (2008) gives an interesting account of this issue in the context of

Southeast Asia. When attempting to collect data on the behaviors and needs of sex workers, researchers found they were missing vital information by limiting demographic choices to boxes labeled "male" and "female," since a significant part of the target population did not identify solely with these titles. Researchers and policy makers interested in an educational response to HIV/AIDS have to increasingly challenge their own assumptions and traditional beliefs about gender and sexuality in order to make their interventions and strategies truly humanitarian.

Transactional sex and sex workers

As with the issue of HIV/AIDS versus HIV and AIDS terminology, accuracy, and sensitivity of language is important to convey both meaning and motive. The term "prostitute" especially has been replaced with the more accurate "sex worker." The phrase "people who exchange sex acts for goods, services, or money," describes the act of *transactional sex*, which does not necessarily come with the identity of "prostitution" ("commercial sex worker" is now considered redundant).

It is vital for researchers and policy makers to take into account sexual activity within the context of transaction. The ability of people to make decisions accordingly and to use knowledge on how to prevent HIV infection (either for themselves or for others) is dependent largely on the power dynamics of not only the coupling, but also the particular event. A woman who identifies herself as a sex worker may be empowered by her identity to require her clients to use condoms as well as having romantic relationships where there is no commercial exchange. In certain political and cultural climates, it might be a better use of scarce resources to empower and support male sex workers to use condoms and get tested rather than attempt to reach other men who have sex with men who do not identify as gay and will not admit to this activity.

While the title of "sex worker" might not be applied to women in forced marriages or younger men and women being supported by *sugar daddies* and *sugar mommies*, researchers and policy makers can use much of the evidence obtained from research on transactional sex. With appropriate modifications, data from this research can help in better understanding the dynamics of an epidemic. Economic independence in this case seems to be one of the defining factors. For people identifying as sex workers, economic security gives them the power to make choices and use what education they have received. For those young people, especially school girls, who are dependent on older men to provide for them, offering alternatives such as free school supplies, uniforms, and transportation and of course tuition can make the difference.

In addition, many women are still sold into marriage. Their families choose the partner based on financial and social reasons, and for women who are of a lower social caste, or have some stigma attached to them because, for example, a family member has HIV/AIDS, or they have a disability, or simply because they are one of many sisters in the family, they will be bought by a much older man who often has other wives and girlfriends. They will have significantly less power in the relationship, be pressured to produce children even at a young age, and live with their new family, away from their birth family and friends. They will have a higher risk of HIV infection, and for lack of treatment, a higher risk of progressing to AIDS and dying. Sex in this relationship may not be completely consensual; instead it may be in exchange for payment to the family, housing, and protection from becoming an outcast. Sex also might be in exchange for not being beaten and emotionally abused, or to ensure wifely status by bearing children. Later in this volume Priya Lall tackles how current HIV/AIDS education between patient and doctor might not always be humanitarian, in that it can often fail to take into consideration these contexts and lose potency.

Concluding remarks on risk groups

The idea of agency and power relations is vital in understanding what terms we use, how they impact what we call a risk group, and who gets targeted with education. Education must match the social, cultural, political, economic, and even biological context of potential infection. It must match which choices the two people have in these situations, and to what extent they can use knowledge to change behavior.

When reading the accounts that this book provides, it is important to remember these issues, especially how in different contexts well-meaning educational programs might backfire and cause greater harm than good. While HIV/AIDS has been around for 30 years, it has largely been seen as a disease of rich, gay Americans. The cultures that are now most affected with this pandemic have had their cultural beliefs and norms established for much, much longer, and there is a real issue of having outsiders, once again, tell them how to live their lives.

HIV/AIDS puts a death marker on these already-strong beliefs about morality and what is proper; it creates a symbol for cultural and social rule breaking and new ways of manifesting the xenophobia for which we all inherently have the potential. When people do not feel they identify with immoral groups and believe they are leading virtuous lives, regardless of their true risk of infection, they will ignore educational messages. This is unfortunately a large problem with monogamous married women who will often say that they are not at risk of HIV, and also very commonly that their faith will protect them. Using risk groups to target educational programs can be extremely useful, but it must be done while taking into consideration the cultural realities, if it is to be successful and not create further harm.

Why hasn't education about these technologies worked so far?

So, if we know how to reduce HIV transmission, if we know what basic technologies impact incidence, why are we seeing *increasing* rates among men who have sex with men in most parts of the world, and more commonly among women in the poorest areas? Why is it that for every single person who starts ART there are at least *three* more who become newly infected? (Cohen et al., 2008). Why aren't we winning the fight in most regions?

These "simple" prevention and treatment methods are not isolated outside the myriad of social, economic, and political struggles within which the HIV epidemic is entrenched. As this book's contributors will discuss in detail in different international contexts, distributing condoms and teaching youth how to use them is an arduous and expensive task, hampered by deep cultural beliefs about their use, gender roles and sexism, religious beliefs, and suspicion and fear about foreign or Western influence. Where the epidemic has reached extreme proportions, as in Eastern and Southern Africa, the local and national health infrastructures, already insufficient to care for their citizens, are even more burdened with large numbers of people who are dying from AIDS-related illnesses

What successes have we seen so far?

The most recent UN reports (UNAIDS, 2010) have indeed shown significant gains, with about 20 percent fewer new infections than a decade earlier, and in the past five years a similar percentage of those infected with HIV have died from AIDS-related illnesses. Since 2001, the rate of new infections has stabilized or decreased including in 34 countries in sub-Saharan Africa. In Ethiopia, South Africa, Zambia, and Zimbabwe rates have decreased by more than 25 percent, while elsewhere in some countries in Eastern Europe and Central Asia, new infections have gone up by as much as 25 percent.

There is some evidence to show that within the most severely affected countries, young people are probably using safer sexual practices. Condom use has increased, and in many countries rates are as high as 75 percent (use at the last higher-risk sexual encounter). Men who have sex with men are also increasingly using condoms, especially in high-risk encounters, and among sex workers, with almost two-thirds of sex workers having used condoms with their most recent client in 69 countries.

While treatment is still inaccessible to the majority of PLWHA (10 million: the number has doubled in only a few years), the total number of people on treatment has increased by 30 percent. There has been an almost 25 percent decrease in HIV transmission to babies from their mothers in the past five years.

Debates over HIV/AIDS education

With so much reliance on the transmission of information to control and mitigate the HIV/AIDS epidemic, it is vital that scarce financial and human resources be efficient and effective. This is a difficult task for many reasons. With decades of efforts and billions of dollars spent, showing little promising results, many researchers are attempting to not only make future interventions better but find out what went wrong in the past.

The debate over "what works"

There is a significant debate over which educational strategies and interventions are effective, centering around a core discussion of what constitutes evidence and how to use it (Piot et al., 2008; Van de Ven and Aggleton, 1999). While everyone agrees that prevention and mitigation through education is vital, and probably the most sustainable and cost-effective way of dealing with HIV/AIDS, not all researchers or policy makers agree on "what works." Researchers and policy makers have recently moved away from describing programs or strategies as "evidence-based" and begun using the phrase "evidence-informed," recognizing the many factors involved in a program's success or failure.

Traditionally randomized controlled trials (RCTs) and systematic reviews are used within the field of medicine to collect data, test hypotheses, and compare results. The outcomes of these trials and reviews are bodies of strong evidence that researchers can use to make claims about new drugs or technologies like the female condom. RCTs are deeply important in determining whether or not a new microbiocide gel actually works across huge samples of thousands of participants, or whether male circumcision actually prevents the spread of HIV. Some researchers, however, critique an over-reliance on these methods or defining "evidence" in general by these parameters. This is especially true when attempting to generalize findings across disparate cultures or communities.

Many researchers are now advocating a balanced approach to the AIDS response, especially in terms of education (Merson et al., 2008). "Evidence-informed" educational programs can include lessons learned from large RCTs conducted in the USA while taking into account the local cultural realities and resource limitations of, for instance, post-earthquake Haiti. Other forms of evidence are increasingly being recognized, especially qualitative studies and what Gupta et al. (2008), call "structural approaches." Much of what authors in this book argue is a humanitarian response falls under this description; educational programs and strategies that seek to change not only individual behaviors but the wider structures (social, political, cultural, economic, even environmental) that impact HIV/AIDS. As David Clarke reminds us in his chapter, local educators and policy makers must "know their epidemic."

This is why a case study, such as that described in Priya Lall's chapter, containing the testimonies of Indian women discussing how they came to know their serostatus, is useful. The same can be said for Fadhila Mazanderani and Jane Anderson's case study of African immigrants in the United Kingdom. The kind of analysis, the questions asked, and answers received from this kind of study are vital in understanding the impact of education that is difficult to include in large RCTs, and cannot be compared easily across large data sets, with systemic reviews. They show how education interacts with HIV/AIDS on a small, very human scale that helps researchers and practitioners begin to ask new questions and modify larger programs in nuanced ways. Education as a humanitarian response in the context of the HIV/AIDS epidemic is as varied as the many communities it affects.

How do HIV and AIDS impact educational institutions, systems and provision?

HIV/AIDS infects families and communities, not just individuals

The presence of HIV/AIDS in a community is like a pebble tossed into a pond. Each person infected, already struggling with stigma and later with the disabling symptoms of AIDS, produces ripples. The economic and social impacts of HIV/AIDS-related stigma and disability is felt strongly by those closest to the individual, but also throughout the ecological networks of their local community, occupation, and country. This is why education as a humanitarian response to this epidemic often addresses more than just individual behavior change, though this is instrumental in impacting the disease. In communities where there is a high prevalence of HIV especially, responses to this disease are increasingly infused into multiple subjects, across most age groups and populations. In these populations, all education can be potentially HIV/AIDS-response education.

Children Orphaned or Made Vulnerable by AIDS

Referring to these children simply as "AIDS orphans" can inaccurately label them as HIV positive as well as increasing stigma, so researchers are now encouraged to reference this population as being orphaned or made vulnerable by AIDS.

Educational responses often focus on the detrimental impact of one or more parent (orphans are so defined by the death of one parent) dying of an AIDS-related illness. Even a family member who is not a parent or primary caregiver having HIV/AIDS can significantly impact the life of a child, especially in terms of education. There are consistent reports of declining school attendance because of a lack of school fees and because children must stay home and care for their parent or family member. These children also face stigma transposed from their infected relatives and are frequently beaten, even by other family members, forced to sell sex to survive and even live on the streets. Because having even one parent die from AIDS is devastating on many levels, these children are included in the definition of *orphan* in this context. Children who are otherwise affected by HIV/AIDS, such as having another family member infected, are considered *vulnerable*. Together, orphans and other vulnerable children, or OVC, are a large focus of the educational response. (For more on how education can help their situation, and how HIV/AIDS impacts their education, see IATTOVC, 2004)

Teachers

In high-prevalence areas where the epidemic is generalized teachers are becoming even more scarce because of AIDS-related deaths. Especially in rural areas, teachers often make comparably higher salaries than most and enjoy greater social status and mobility, all factors that lead to riskier sexual behavior. Some research has shown that this situation has led to a greater likelihood of contiguous relationships alongside marriage, a perfect transmitter for the virus, to the point that teachers are themselves considered a high-risk group in some areas. In Zambia, for instance, the rate of AIDS deaths among teachers is 70 percent higher than for the general population. In South Africa, the rate of HIV infection among teachers is 20–30 percent (Carr-Hill, et al., 2002).

Teacher productivity is also affected by the disabling aspects of AIDS. Government reporting of the actual teaching hours lost, whether due to AIDS-related illnesses or other reasons, is scarce, but given the number of teachers reported dying from AIDS we can project the numbers. Based on the viral timeline, without treatment, AIDS-related death is preceded by about 18 months of significant disability, where teachers are less attentive to their classes or fail to show at all. During the last six months to one year of AIDS before death, it is probable that no meaningful teaching is occurring at all. In addition, especially in the case of female teachers, if a family member is dying from AIDS, the teacher will need to stay home to care for that relative, foregoing her classes.

Research has also shown that male teachers frequently cultivate sexual relationships with female students, often in exchange for school fees, high marks, or other goods or services. Younger females are frequently viewed by these older men as safer, clean, and uninfected, and so an entire generation of HIV-positive men, the large majority of whom are not aware of their serostatus, are infecting a generation of younger women and girls. There is also the issue of rape and abuse between teachers/educators and students as many of these "relationships" are not consensual. These cases are arguably higher in boarding schoolings, which for many populations are a common educational choice.

As education is increasingly being seen as a panacea or "vaccine" for many problems, namely HIV/AIDS, teachers are under great pressure to include more and more topics in their instruction, which they often have little or no additional training for. The frequently mandated HIV/AIDS education curriculum in most schools, though ideally an efficient way of getting to the wider population in generalized epidemics, is often viewed with skepticism, anxiety, and frustration by teachers. Without adequate training and support, teachers report negative attitudes to talking to their students about sex because of social taboos, especially, and will change the curriculum or avoid teaching the subject entirely. This is especially true when teachers are under the pressure of high-stakes testing, used to evaluate teacher and school performance, and when classroom time and teacher energy is limited. Religious and cultural beliefs of teachers are often not addressed by international or domestic agencies mandating HIV/AIDS education, with discussion of condoms being especially problematic for teachers. While this can be managed with adequate training and support, it should be recognized that teachers undergo added stresses when they and their students are living with a generalized epidemic.

Costs of schooling

It is important to understand the culture around education in more resource-poor settings in terms of how HIV/AIDS impacts entire communities. Losing a parent or having to pay for treatment can result in school being a financial, social, and even practical impossibility. While universal primary education is a goal worldwide and *technically* available in most countries, there are often hidden or implicit costs. Individual schools and teachers may charge students because their own salaries and funding may not be enough to continue adequate schooling. Paper, writing instruments, chalk, chairs, and books, especially, are usually not provided and must be bought by students. In many rural settings the cost of a textbook will be equal to a week or more of pay, if the book is even available for purchase in the area, which is also rare. There are few libraries, bookstores, or other places to buy school supplies, and maintenance of schools can also be costly and not always supported by the government. Wearing a school uniform, even when not required, is culturally a necessity, and children will often stay home from school if they cannot afford a uniform. To avoid this issue in some countries, free uniforms have begun to be distributed to children when they enroll at their local school.

The role of schools

More distal effects on education can be seen in looking at the political and economic results of HIV/AIDS as a generalized epidemic. Schools are increasingly serving as more than educational institutions, with orphans and HIV-positive students requiring services and support. They have become gateways for treatment and other medical services as well as food and nutrition; for many, school is where students will have their only guaranteed meal of the day. As teacher shortages are combined with an ever-increasing push for education for all, more students than ever are showing up for school in crowded classrooms with sometimes 100 students per teacher. With teacher shortages, the likelihood of complete and sufficient training is slim. In short, HIV/AIDS puts enormous pressures on schools and teachers to do more with less. (For a comprehensive review of the effects of HIV/AIDS on schooling including statistics on these issues, see Kelly, 2000)

Conclusion

I introduced this overview by referencing several important themes that are often lost in the machine of HIV/AIDS research and policy: namely the very real people who deal with these issues daily. The epidemic, as this book is being written, is almost 30 years old. While the history of this virus can be traced decades earlier, it was only in 1981 that it received a name, and the idea of AIDS and HIV was truly born. There is an entire generation of people who have no memory of a world without AIDS, without red ribbons, and fundraisers, and calls to action. The future of HIV/AIDS research, policy, and practice will be made possible by these new generations, who have always lived with HIV/AIDS as part of their world, and which directly interact with it in more ways than ever.

I intentionally made reference to recent developments in internet-based communications because while these were once considered only novelties, social networking sites, SMS, smart phones, and other new technologies are now being used for education about HIV/AIDS. Websites and search engines, as explored by Mazanderandi and Anderson's chapter, are complementing and even taking the place of traditional person-to-person education. The internet is a also a place to avoid the stigma of being HIV-positive, or to ask questions about this disease, the place where people can anonymously gather to share stories or simply read and learn about how their lives are not abnormal, how their experiences are very much the experiences of millions worldwide. Researchers and practitioners are experimenting with new ways of using cell phones, which have rapidly become popular even in the poorest areas of the world, to help patients adhere to treatment schedules and obtain information on mobile clinics, or simply to remind people of safer sex practices.

These new possibilities require thinking about education as more than something that happens between teachers and students in a classroom at a school. Those who study education and social science perspectives on learning and information exchange have a great deal to offer the field of HIV/AIDS education, and not just the effects of HIV/AIDS on education, as has been more the tradition. This is not to say, of course, that those in public health and medicine do not or cannot hold such points of view, as in many cases they do. But it is important sometimes to have people who take great stock in social theories and methods help answer the many questions we still have. HIV is a disease, but it is one transmitted, primarily, through the most intimate of social acts between two people who are seeking a social connection if their act is consensual. For medicine to help it must be consciously practiced for people living in an ecological network of cultures, languages, political and economic realities and even environmental and geographic contexts. HIV/AIDS is now part of that network, and if we are to succeed in reducing rates of infection and making the lives of those who are HIV-positive better, we need to consider this network, and only artificially separate out variables when absolutely necessary.

Reference list

Allen, T., and Heald, S. (2004). "HIV/AIDS policy in Africa: what has worked in Uganda and what has failed in Botswana?" *Journal of International Development* 16: 1141–54.

Auvert, B. D. Taljaard, E. Lagarde, J. Sobngwi-Tambekou, R. Sitta and A. Puren. (2005) "Randomized, controlled intervention trial of male circumcision for reduction of HIV infection risk: the ANRS 1265 trial." *PLoS Med* 2: e298.

Bailey R., R. C. Bailey, S. Moses, C. B. Parker, K. Agot, I. Maclean, J. N. Krieger, C. F. Williams, R. T. Campbell and J. O. Ndinya-Achola. (2007). "Male circumcision for HIV prevention in young men in Kisumu, Kenya: a randomized controlled trial." *Lancet* 369: 643–56.

Basuki, E., I. Wolffers, W. Deville, N. Erlaini, D. Luhpuri, R. Hargano, N. Maskuri, N. Suesen and N. van Beelen. (2002). "Reasons for not using condoms among female sex workers in Indonesia." *AIDS Education and Prevention* 14 (2): 102–16

Biggs, N. A. (2010). "Adapting HIV/AIDS education for Deaf Kenyans and the impact of local context." Presentation at the XVIII International AIDS Conference, Vienna, Austria (July 23).

Burke, J. (2004). "Infant HIV infection: acceptability of preventive strategies in central Tanzania." *AID Education and Prevention* 16 (5): 415–25.

Carr-Hill, R., K. J. Katabaro, A. R. Katahoire, and D. Oulai. (2002). *The Impact of HIV/AIDS on education and institutionalizing preventive education.* Published in the series *Education in the Context of HIV/AIDS.* Paris: UNESCO.

Cohen, M. S., N. Hellmann, J. A. Levy, K. Decock and J. Lange. (2008). "The spread, treatment, and prevention of HIV-1: evolution of a global pandemic." *The Journal of Clinical Investigation* 1(18): 1244–54.

Cornman, D. H., S. M. Kiene, S. Christie, W. A. Fisher, P. A. Shuper, S. Pillay, G. H. Friedland, C. M. Thomas, L. Lodge, and J. D. Fisher. (2008). "Clinic-based intervention reduces unprotected sexual behavior among HIV-infected patients in KwaZulu-Natal, South Africa: results of a pilot study." *Journal of Acquired Immune Deficiency Syndromes* 48(5), 553–60.

Donnell, D., J. Kiarie, K. Thomas, J. Baeten, J. Lingappa, C. Cohen, and C. Celum. (2010). "ART and risk of heterosexual HIV-1 transmission in HIV-1 serodiscordant African couples: a multinational prospective study." [Abstract # 136]. 17th Conference on Retroviruses and Opportunistic Infections (CROI); San Francisco, USA.

Dosekun, O., and J. Fox. (2010). "An overview of the relative risks of different sexual behaviours on HIV transmission." *Current Opinion in HIV and AIDS* 5 (4): 291–7.

Fox, J., and S. Fidler. (2010). "Sexual transmission of HIV-1." *Antiviral Research* 85(1): 276–85.

Gilbert, P., D. Ciccarone, S. A. Gansky, D. R. Bangsberg, K. Clanon, S. J. McPhee, S. H. Calderon, A. Bogetz, and B. Gerbert. (2008). "Interactive 'video-doctor' counseling reduces drug and sexual risk behaviors among HIV-positive patients in diverse outpatient settings." *PLoS One* 3: e88.

Gray, R. H., G. Kigozi, D. Serwadda, F. Makumbi, S. Watya, F. Nalugoda, N. Kiwanuka, L. H. Moulton, M. A. Chaudhary, M. Z. Chen, N. K. Sewankambo, F. Wabwire-Mangen, M. C. Bacon, C. F. M. Williams, P. Opendi, S. J. Reynolds, O. Laeyendecker, T. C. Quinn, and M. J. Wawer. (2007). "Male circumcision for HIV prevention in men in Rakai, Uganda: a randomized trial." *The Lancet* 369: 657–66.

Groce, N., and R. Trasi. (2004). "Rape of individuals with disability: AIDS and the folk belief of virgin cleansing." *The Lancet* 363:1663–4.

Gupta, G. R., J. O. Parkhurst, J. A. Ogden, P. Aggleton, and A. Mahal. (2008). "Structural approaches to HIV prevention." *The Lancet* 372: 764–75.

Halperin, D. (2009). "Combination HIV prevention must be based on evidence." *The Lancet* 373: 544–5.

Halperin, D., M. J. Steiner, M. M. Cassell, E. C. Green, N. Hearst, D. Kirby, H. D. Gayle, and W. Cates. (2004). "Time has come for common ground on preventing sexual transmission of HIV." *The Lancet* 364: 1913.

Imgram, B., D. Flannery, A. Elkavich, and M. Rotheram-Borus. (2008). "Common processes in evidence-based adolescent HIV prevention programs." *AIDS Behavior* 12: 374–83.

Inter Agency Task Team on Education, Orphans and Vulnerable Children (IATTEOVC) (2004). *The Role of Education in the Protection, Care and Support of Orphans and Vulnerable Children Living in a World with HIV and AIDS.* Geneva: UNAIDS.

Kalichman, S. (2008). "Time to take stock in HIV/AIDS prevention." *AIDS Behavior* 12: 333–4 .

Kelly, M. J. (2000). *Planning for Education in the Context of HIV/AIDS.* In *Fundamentals of Education Planning*, 6. Paris: International Institute for Education Planning, UNESCO.

Kenyon, C., S. Dlamini, A. Boulle, R. G. White, and M. Badri. (2009). "A network-level explanation for the differences in HIV prevalence in South Africa's racial groups." *African Journal of AIDS Research* 3: 243–54.

Macintyre, K., L. Brown, and S. Sosler. (2001). " 'It's not what you know, but who you knew': examining the relationship between behavior change and AIDS mortality in Africa." *AIDS Education and Prevention* 13 (2): 160–74.

Marks, G., N. Crepaz, and R. S. Janssen. (2006). "Estimating sexual transmission of HIV from persons aware and unaware that they are infected with the virus in the USA." *AIDS* 20: 1447–50

Merson, M., J. O'Malley, D. Serwadda, and C. Apisuk. (2008). "The history and challenge of HIV Prevention." *The Lancet* 372: 475–88.

Merson, M., N. Pandian, T. J. Coates, G. R. Gupta, S. M. Bertozzi, P. Pilot, P. Mane, and M. Bartos. (2008). "Combination HIV prevention." *The Lancet* 372: 1805–6.

Pantaleo, G., C. Graziosi, and A. S. Fauci. (1993). "New concepts in the immunopathogenesis of human immunodeficiency virus infection." *New England Journal of Medicine* 328 (5): 327–35.

Parkhurst, J. (2002). "The Ugandan success story? Evidence and claims of HIV-1 prevention." *The Lancet* 360: 78–80.

Piot, P., M. Bartos, H. Larson, D. Zewdie, and P. Mane. (2008). "Coming to terms with complexity: a call to action for HIV prevention." *The Lancet* 372: 845–59.

Pisani, E. (2008). *The Wisdom of Whores.* London: Granta Books.

Rosenstock, I. M. (1974). *Historical Origins of the Health Belief Model.* Health Education Monographs 2, New Jersey: Prentice Hall.

Schaalma, H., L. E. Aaro, A. J. Flisher, C. Mathews, S. Kaaya, H. Onya, A. Ragnarson, and K. Klepp. (2009). "Correlates of intention to use condoms among sub-Saharan African youth: the applicability of the theory of planned behaviour." *Scandinavian Journal of Public Health* 37 (2 Suppl.): 87–91.

Thomson S. C., W. Ombidi, C. Toroitich-Ruto, E. L. Wong, H. O. Tucker, R. Homan, N. Kingola, and S. Luchters. (2006). "A prospective study assessing the effects of Kenya introducing the female condom in a sex worker population in Mombasa, Kenya." *Sexually Transmitted Infections*, 82: 397–407.

UNAIDS (2008). *Report on the Global HIV/AIDS Epidemic.* Geneva: UNAIDS.

— (2009). *UNAIDS Newsletter/09: No Single Magic Bullet for HIV Prevention.* Geneva: UNAIDS.

— (2010). *Report on the Global AIDS Epidemic 2010*. Geneva: UNAIDS.

Van de Ven, P. and P. Aggleton. (1999). "What constitutes evidence in HIV/AIDS education?" *Health Education Research* 14 (4): 461–71.

Vernazza, P., B. Hirschel, E. Bernasconi, and M. Flepp. (2008). "HIV transmission under highly active antiretroviral therapy." *The Lancet,* 372: 1806.

F. Veronese, P. Anton, C. Fletcher, V. DeGruttola, I. McGowan, S. Becker, S. Zwerski, and D. Burns. (2010). "Implications of HIV PrEP Trials Results." *AIDS Research and Human Retroviruses,* 27 (1): 81–90.

Volk, J. F. and C. Koopman. (2001). "Factors associated with condom use in Kenya: a test of the health belief model." *AIDS Education and Prevention* 13 (6): 495–508.

Wawer, M. J., R. H. Gray, N. K. Sewankambo, D. Serwadda, X. Li, O. Laeyendecker, N. Kiwanuka, G. Kigozi, M. Kiddugavu, T. Lutalo, F. Nalugoda, F. Wabwire-Mangen, M. P. Meehan, T. C. Quinn. (2005). "Rates of HIV-1 transmission per coital act, by stage of HIV-1 infection, in Rakai, Uganda." *Journal of Infectious Diseases* 1: 1403–9.

West, G., A. L. Corneli, K. Best, K. M. Kurkjian, and W. Cates Jr. (2007). "Focusing HIV prevention on those most likely to transmit the virus." *AIDS Education & Prevention* 19 (4): 275–88

World Health Organization (WHO) (2008) *Towards Universal Access: Scaling up Priority HIV/AIDS Interventions in the Health Sector.* Geneva: WHO.

— (2009). *Rapid Advice: Antiretroviral Therapy for HIV Infection in Adults and Adolescents.* Geneva: WHO.

Yankah, E., and P. Aggleton (2008). "Effects and effectiveness of life skills education for HIV prevention in young people." *AIDS Education & Prevention* 20 (6): 465–85.

Yotebieng, M., C. T. Halpern, E. M. H. Mitchell, and A. A. Adimora, (2009). "Correlates of condom use among sexually experienced secondary-school male students in Nairobi, Kenya." *SAHARA J: Journal of Social Aspects of HIV/AIDS Research Alliance* 6 (1): 9–16.

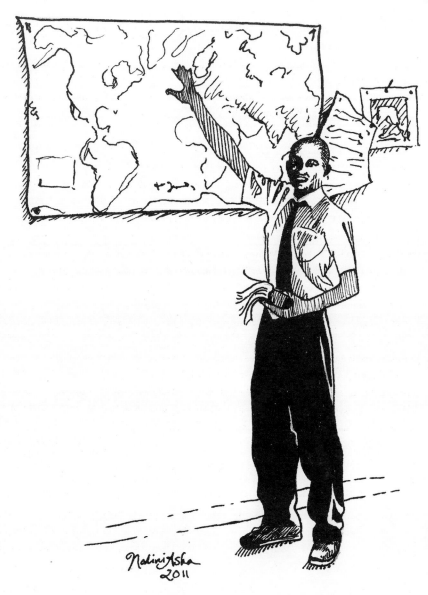

Young Deaf man, about to graduate from secondary school in western Kenya, by Nalini Asha Biggs, Pen and Ink, 2011

International Responses to HIV/AIDS and Education

Christopher Castle and Mark Richmond

1

Chapter Outline

Introduction

Recent data show that the number of new HIV infections is steadily falling or leveling off in most parts of the world. Between 2001 and 2009, 22 countries in sub-Saharan Africa saw a decline of more than 25 percent in new HIV infections. Some of the countries with the most severe epidemics in Africa—namely, Côte d'Ivoire, Ethiopia, Nigeria, South Africa, Zambia, and Zimbabwe—are leading the way in reducing new HIV infections and are making real progress toward achieving Target 6a of Millennium Development Goal 6 (MDG 6): to halt and begin to reverse the spread of HIV by 2015. In addition, worldwide there are now 5.2 million people on antiretroviral therapy (ART), which represents a twelvefold increase in six years. As a result, in 2008 there were 200,000 *fewer* AIDS-related deaths than in 2004. Owing to wide-scale prevention efforts, young people are having sex later, having fewer partners, and using condoms, resulting in significantly fewer new HIV infections in many of those countries highly affected by AIDS.

These new figures represent grounds for hope and optimism and are a testament to concerted international, national, and civil-society response efforts. They also demonstrate how individuals around the world, and especially young people, are taking proactive measures to protect themselves from HIV infection as well as challenging traditional social values and gender norms. Nevertheless, many challenges and implementation bottlenecks still remain. Since 2001, HIV prevalence in Russia, Eastern Europe, and Central Asia has approximately doubled, making the regions home to the world's most rapidly expanding epidemic. Meanwhile, in several high-income countries, there has been a resurgence of HIV infections among men who have sex with men (MSM). Although access to treatment has been massively scaled up, out of the estimated 33 million people living with HIV in the world, only about one person in three needing ART in low- and middle-income countries receives it. In many sub-Saharan African countries, this figure is less than one in four. Moreover, there are still huge numbers of children and young people who do not have access to correct information about HIV prevention and have not acquired the values and skills necessary to protect themselves. If development goals and targets are to be met, the international community must build on these jointly won gains and ensure that efforts are sustained and expanded.

The need for a comprehensive approach

Over the course of the epidemic, the response to HIV/AIDS has changed significantly. In the early years, HIV and AIDS were considered to be a medical problem associated with certain so-called high-risk groups such as injecting drug users, men who have sex with men, as well as contaminated blood. Consequently, the initial response was chiefly led by the World Health Organization (WHO). As the epidemic became more generalized and prevalence rates soared, particularly in sub-Saharan African countries, the international community recognized that HIV and AIDS were no longer solely a public health crisis but also a large-scale development crisis. As the epidemic worsened, many hard-won development gains were eroded or threatened. This is because HIV/AIDS reduces life expectancy, increases child mortality, leaves large numbers of children without adult care, places extra burdens on health-care systems, negatively affects economic development, and impoverishes households. HIV/AIDS also exacerbates the underlying conditions that drive development, such as education (Kelly, 2000). The education sector is significant in that it can positively affect a country's socioeconomic viability and has access to a ready-made infrastructure for delivering prevention programs to children and young people (World Bank, 2002).

However, formal education is particularly vulnerable to HIV/AIDS, given the extremely human-resource-intensive nature of the sector. It has been estimated that between one-fifth and one-quarter of the world's population works in formal education-related jobs or is in at least part-time schooling, and so has a daily and intimate relationship with the sector. HIV/AIDS impacts all aspects of education by reducing the demand for, supply of, and quality of, education. Fewer children attend school as they become ill or are required to stay at home to care for sick relatives. Other children are taken out of school to engage in income-generating activities as already-scarce household resources are diverted to health-care. In most cases, already-vulnerable children such as girls or children with disabilities are the first to lose educational opportunities. On the supply side, trained educators are lost through mortality and sickness, and many teachers migrate to towns and cities in order to access health-care facilities that are not available in rural areas. Others, both educators and learners, leave formal schooling because they are quite simply unable to cope with the stigma and discrimination they face in the school or the community.

In terms of quality, classes may be interrupted or not take place at all, with experienced teachers being replaced with less well-trained teachers—if they are replaced at all. The results are reduced efficiency, productivity, and achievement throughout the entire education system. Other sectors, already overburdened and struggling to meet national needs and internationally set development goals, take on these extra challenges and the effects pan out on many levels.

Because HIV/AIDS has impacted those very institutions, such as education, that would otherwise drive development, there has been a growing recognition within the international community that a multisectoral approach is necessary, one that involves a variety of actors and stakeholders with different areas of technical expertize working together. Therefore in 1996, the Joint United Nations Programme on HIV and AIDS (UNAIDS) was launched to strengthen and consolidate the way in which the United Nations (UN) responded to HIV/AIDS.

UNAIDS is guided by a Programme Coordinating Board with representatives of 22 governments, 10 UN organizations, which are referred to as the cosponsors, and 5 representatives of nongovernmental organizations (NGOs) including associations of people living with HIV. A series of goals, resolutions and declarations adopted by UN member states established a framework within which the international community could work toward halting and reversing the spread of HIV and scaling up to achieve universal access to prevention programs, treatment, care, and support. UNAIDS believes that achieving universal access will help reach target 6a of the MDG (to halt and reverse the spread of HIV) as well as have a significant impact on broader health and development goals such as maternal mortality, poverty and gender equality. It is important to bear in mind that all the MDGs are interlinked and mutually reinforcing, thus addressing HIV helps to achieve all the MDGs.

UNAIDS, comprised of the cosponsors and the Secretariat, is active in a variety of areas such as advocacy, strengthening leadership, building the evidence base to support programs, supporting the use of strategic information, setting standards and norms, and providing technical support to countries to assist them in the implementation of their national AIDS plans. Under the UNAIDS "division of labour," (which is currently being revised to reflect the changing nature of the epidemic and hence the response), each cosponsor is designated as the lead organization in a specific area, based on its comparative advantage.

Thus, the United Nations Educational, Scientific and Cultural Organization (UNESCO) has been the lead organization for HIV prevention with young people in educational institutions. This designation of lead organizations aims to assist UNAIDS in delivering unified and consolidated support at the country level throughout its program, and to avoid duplication and fragmentation. The lead organization acts as a single entry point for government and other country-level stakeholders requiring support within a particular area. It is also largely responsible for coordinating the provision and facilitation of this support, which generally takes the form of expertize but increasingly involves assisting countries to plan ahead and predict what they are going to need for different aspects of their HIV/AIDS responses. Moreover, the lead organization acts as a liaison between UNAIDS and other providers of support in its area, as well as between UN Theme Groups and global support mechanisms. The majority of funding for UNAIDS comes from bilateral donors (UN member states), certain cosponsors, and other funding mechanisms such as private foundations.

Duplication, fragmentation, and competition for funding are criticisms that often have been leveled at UN organizations. In 2005, to respond to these and other challenges as well as promote strengthened coherence and coordination, the Secretary-General's High-Level Panel on UN System-wide Coherence recommended the One UN initiative: one leader, one program, one budget, and one office. Later characterized as Delivering as One, this initiative aims to ensure faster and more effective development operations and accelerate progress toward achieving the MDGs by establishing a consolidated UN presence while building on the strengths and comparative advantages of the different members of the UN family. The initiative has been piloted in eight countries: Albania, Cape Verde, Mozambique, Pakistan, Rwanda, Tanzania, Uruguay, and Viet Nam.

In terms of the education sector, these coherence and coordination reforms have given the sector valuable traction by ensuring that education is not isolated but instead is fully mainstreamed into UN-wide comprehensive responses to HIV/AIDS. Harnessing multisectoral approaches is seen as essential in responding to complex issues like HIV/AIDS. In addition, the regular interaction and exchanges between UN agencies and the cosponsors helps position education as an integral part of an ongoing process. While there are still many challenges ahead, it is an example of how the One UN concept is starting to become a reality.

Contributing to these reforms, efforts to increase collaboration, encourage technical exchanges, and promote interagency harmonization and coordination were already being implemented through the establishment of interagency task teams (IATTs). The UNAIDS IATT on Education, which is convened by UNESCO, was created in 2002 to support accelerated and improved education-sector responses to HIV/AIDS. The main goals of the UNAIDS IATT on Education are promoting and supporting good practices related to HIV/AIDS in the education sector and encouraging alignment and harmonization within and across agencies to support global and country-level actions. It is distinctive in that its members include not only UNAIDS cosponsors but also bilateral agencies, private foundations, and civil-society organizations involved in supporting education-sector responses to HIV/AIDS.

Shared leadership and membership engagement underpin the IATT, reflected in the structure of the Steering Committee and Working Groups, and in particular in the rotational hosting of the biannual meetings. Within the IATT on Education, there are currently five Working Groups, and these cover issues including higher education, indicators, and education in emergencies. Working groups also provide technical support and inputs into important initiatives such as the Education for All Fast Track Initiative (EFA FTI) and the *EFA Global Monitoring Report*. In 2002, the IATT on Education established the Accelerate Initiative Working Group to support countries in sub-Saharan Africa to accelerate their education sector responses to HIV/AIDS. The working group organized a series of subregional workshops where participants included representatives of the education sector (including formal and informal subsectors) and teachers' associations. The aims of the workshops were twofold: first, to create common understanding of the role that the education sector could play in responding to HIV and AIDS, and, second, to encourage sectoral leadership and action at the country level. Over the past five years, four networks of HIV and AIDS Focal Points have been set up throughout Africa and have taken on responsibility and ownership of the Accelerate activities at regional and national levels (Bundy et al., 2007).

A key aspect of the IATT's work is to strengthen the evidence base on HIV/AIDS and education and disseminate findings to inform decision making and strategy development, which it does through the production of documents and tools. In 2004, the IATT conducted the first international baseline survey, titled *Global HIV/AIDS Readiness Survey*, to investigate the capacity and readiness of countries to manage the impact of HIV/AIDS on their education systems. In addition, it intended to help participating countries better identify key problems and omissions in their response, and guide future planning and programming. Although the survey found that 72 percent of participating ministries had management structures or committees to guide the sector's response, these structures were often weak and overburdened. The exercise was valuable insofar as the survey inputs have been used to hold ministries accountable for their stated commitments. Partial funding has recently been secured to carry out a follow-up survey, titled *Global Progress Survey*, which will measure what has happened since the first survey was conducted, identify trends, and explore in greater depth some of the challenges and bottlenecks affecting the implementation of good-quality HIV prevention education within educational institutions and processes.

In 2010, the IATT published *Updated Stocktaking Report: Education Sector Responses to HIV and AIDS*, which included an extensive literature review—first carried out in 2009—on research on HIV/AIDS in the education sector. The report identifies research carried out by the IATT, its members and others, and draws attention to gaps in and ways of complementing and building upon existing research. The report covers four areas: HIV prevention; education and HIV mitigation; the impact of education on demand and supply of education; and policy responses. In 2010, the IATT published a companion piece to the stocktaking report entitled the *Quality of Evidence Assessment for Literature Considering the Impact of Education on HIV and AIDS*, which provides an in-depth analysis of the data collected through the stocktaking review of research on HIV/AIDS in the education sector carried out by the Overseas Development Institute (ODI). It provides a summary of the quality and type of evidence available on the impact of education on HIV and AIDS responses, indicating strengths and weaknesses, in order to make suggestions for future research.

Another important UNAIDS initiative, which seeks to promote coordination and strengthen the evidence base, is the Global Initiative on Education and HIV & AIDS, or EDUCAIDS. Launched in 2004, it is a multicountry initiative led by UNESCO. EDUCAIDS is central to contributing to a strong national response to HIV/AIDS, as well to achieving the EFA goals and the MDGs. The two main objectives of EDUCAIDS are to prevent the spread of HIV through education and to protect the core functions of the education systems from the worst effects of the epidemic. EDUCAIDS differs from the IATT on Education in that it is country led and country driven. Although the IATT seeks to promote good practice and to improve alignment and harmonization at the country level, it does not in itself act as an "organization" supporting long-term and sustained country-level action. This is the responsibility of the agencies/initiatives that are affiliated with the IATT, of which EDUCAIDS is one (UNESCO, 2006).

EDUCAIDS has produced a Framework for Action to improve understanding of the need for strong education-sector engagement in national HIV/AIDS responses as part of efforts toward universal access. EDUCAIDS assists partners to identify actions needed at the country level to address the epidemic in a comprehensive and effective manner. Fundamental to this approach is the delivery of a joint partner/stakeholder situation and needs analysis at the country level. This analysis focuses on identifying which elements of an effective response are in place and which need to be developed. The assessment is then used to develop a strategy for addressing the identified gaps, supporting governments and partners to scale up the response to HIV and AIDS, and mobilizing resources to address the identified priorities. EDUCAIDS promotes a comprehensive approach based on a framework of five interrelated components, namely: 1) quality education; 2) content, curriculum, and learning materials; 3) educator training and support; 4) approaches and illustrative entry points; and 5) policy, management, and systems. EDUCAIDS' philosophy is that these five components need to be in place and working well to ensure optimal success in the educational response to the epidemic.

EDUCAIDS has produced a resource pack, which contains the Framework for Action, an Overview of Practical Resources (documents, toolkits, etc.) and 35 Technical Briefs. The briefs are two-page summaries of key issues related to the aforementioned five components. The resource pack is intended for officials in ministries of education and other organizations supporting the development and implementation of policies, determining resources, and implementing programs for education sector staff and learners.

Since it was established, 53 countries in five regions have engaged with EDUCAIDS. To describe progress and lessons learned, EDUCAIDS produces a series of "country snapshots." In Viet Nam, for example, the UN family worked together to support the country's education sector response to HIV/AIDS by strengthening institutional structures and mechanisms in its Ministry of Education and Training (MOET), supporting strategic planning and inclusion of HIV/AIDS and sexuality education in national strategy documents; supporting the monitoring and evaluation of HIV/AIDS education; and advocating for inclusion of HIV prevention in the education sector. In terms of lessons learned, it is clear that for advocacy efforts to be successful, UN agencies must continue to work together to ensure coordinated action and maximum impact. EDUCAIDS provided a clear framework for the UN Education Sub-Group in its support to the MOET. It was also used to assist in the development of the MOET's proposal to the Global Fund to Fight AIDS, Tuberculosis and Malaria (GFATM). Coordination through these various mechanisms was enhanced by Viet Nam's status as a One UN pilot country, which also allowed it to benefit from One Plan funds and other resources.

In 2008, an independent evaluation of EDUCAIDS commissioned by UNESCO found that, on the whole, progress had been made by the education sector in its response to HIV/AIDS and was particularly strong in the areas of policy development, planning, coordination, integration of HIV/AIDS in secondary education curricula, and care and support for learners. In some countries, EDUCAIDS was found to have made a contribution to the education sector response through the provision of resources, reinforcing coordination mechanisms, sharing and promoting best practices, and strengthening the evidence base.

Evidence-based approaches

Evidence-based approaches are critical to delivering relevant comprehensive education sector prevention responses; for this reason, UNAIDS, EDUCAIDS, the IATT on Education, the cosponsors and other education partners place great importance on undertaking, commissioning, and actively disseminating research on wide-ranging aspects of HIV/AIDS and education. The findings of these studies and surveys are used to increase the knowledge base, identify best practices, and inform policies. However, due to the changing course of the epidemic and the emergence of local challenges, there is a continued need for up-to-date research and data on changes in trends. This is essential because what was true ten years ago is not necessarily true today and responses must be able to reflect this if they are to be effective.

A good example of the need to regularly monitor trends was revealed in a study on the relationship between HIV infection and educational status. A meta-analysis of 36 studies carried out in 11 sub-Saharan countries between 1987 and 2003 found that studies prior to 1996 generally found either no association between educational status and HIV risk or found that the highest risk was among the most educated; by contrast, data collected after 1996 have tended to find a lower risk among the most educated (Hargreaves et al., 2008). Further research suggests that remaining in school longer, over and above any specific prevention programs, helps reduce the risks and rates of infection and can also respond to the additional needs of children infected and affected by HIV/AIDS. It is believed that this is most likely because education promotes a number of factors that can reduce vulnerability to HIV infection such as equipping young people with literacy skills in order to read information, developing decision making and critical thinking skills, promoting self-confidence and coping skills, and contributing to postponing the age of sexual debut. It also empowers girls, which is especially important as two-thirds of newly infected young people aged 15–19 are female. Studies have shown that girls who have completed secondary education have a lower risk of HIV infection (Hargreaves et al., 2006). A study conducted in Zimbabwe found that the HIV prevalence among 15–18 year old girls who had remained in school was 1.3 percent compared to 7.2 percent in girls of the same age group who had dropped out of school (ActionAid International and Save the Children Fund, UK, 2004).

An initiative to keep girls in school has been piloted by the World Bank and it has recently released a study on the initiative entitled *Schooling, Income, and HIV Risk*. The study, which was conducted in Malawi between 2008 and 2009, randomly selected 3,796 girls and young women between the ages of 13 and 22 from Zomba, a district with high HIV infection and school dropout rates among adolescent girls. The only condition for receiving cash payments was that the girls enrolled in the program had to attend school on a regular basis. Eighteen months after the program began, it was found that HIV infections among girls in the program were 60 percent lower than those who were part of the control group, which did not receive payments.

Prevention programs

In addition to remaining in school longer, young people also have access to comprehensive prevention programs to further reduce new infections. However, comprehensive and correct knowledge of HIV/AIDS among young people is still unacceptably low in many countries and less than one-third of young men and less than one-fifth of young women in developing countries have satisfactory knowledge (United Nations, 2010). These levels fall far short of the target, established at the 2006 UN General Assembly Special Session on HIV and AIDS (UNGASS), of 95 percent by 2010. Acquiring this knowledge is critical as young people aged 15–24 account for 45 percent of all new HIV infections (UNAIDS, 2008).

While ministries of education have given considerable attention to curriculum development and many countries do now include HIV/AIDS education in their curricula, quality is varied and evaluations have found that this education tends to focus almost exclusively on knowledge and facts, with little or no attention given to attitudes, values, and behaviors. Characteristics of more successful programs include targeting younger students, longer program duration, the use of participatory activities, and the utilization of both peer educators and teachers (Gallant and Maticka-Tyndale, 2004). A recent report published by UNICEF found that progress has been made in preventing new HIV infections among young people aged 15–24 and that in countries where declines in prevalence have been noted they have been most marked among young people. However, the study also found that no single prevention strategy has proved optimal in all circumstances and many young people remain vulnerable to HIV infection (UNICEF et al., 2010).

In 2009, UNESCO collaborated with UNAIDS, UNFPA, UNICEF and WHO to prepare and publish a report entitled *International Technical Guidance on Sexuality Education: An Evidence-informed Approach for Schools, Teachers and Health Educators*. This two-volume document explores the rationale for sexuality education and provides technical advice on what constitutes an effective program as well as guidance on the topics and learning objectives to be covered in four distinct age ranges. Since HIV is primarily sexually transmitted, young people need to be provided with age-appropriate, culturally relevant, and scientifically accurate information about sex and relationships, as well as help in acquiring the necessary skills and values to make responsible choices about when, if, and under what circumstances they decide to have sexual intercourse. This is a challenging area and one that can meet with resistance. A common concern about the provision of sexuality education is that it can lead to early sex. However, extensive research demonstrates that this is seldom the case. In fact, sexuality education can lead to delayed sexual debut and more responsible sexual behavior (Kirby, 2007).

Another concern is that sexuality education goes against cultural and religious norms. Consequently, *International Technical Guidance* stresses the importance of cultural relevance and local implementation by building support with cultural and religious leaders in the community. Key stakeholders must be involved in developing what form sexuality education takes if it is to be accepted. *International Technical Guidance* also stresses the importance of changing social norms and harmful practices (e.g., forced marriages) that are not in line with human rights and increase vulnerability and risk, especially for girls and young women. It is vital that sex education fully addresses gender norms and inequality in terms of how these affect sexuality, behavior, and reproductive health. Gender discrimination is widespread and young women often have little power or control in their relationships, making them more vulnerable to abuse and exploitation. It is worth mentioning that gender norms about men and masculinity—which often have adverse effects for women and girls—also often have adverse effects for men and boys.

The *International Technical Guidance* aims to ensure that the topics and learning objectives address children and young people's need for information. Some of the learning objectives have been specifically designed to reduce unsafe sexual behavior while others focus on increasing awareness and knowledge, and changing social norms. If implemented with good quality and on a large-scale basis, sex education can contribute toward achieving the MDGs and in particular MDG 3 (achieving gender equality and empowerment of women), MDG 5 (reducing maternal mortality and achieving universal access to reproductive health) and MDG 6 (combating HIV/AIDS).

In 2008, the Commission on AIDS in Asia report, entitled *Redefining AIDS in Asia: Crafting an Effective Response*, found that 95 percent of all HIV infections in Asia are driven by three key behaviors: unprotected sex in the context of sex work; unsafe injection of drugs; and unprotected (mainly anal) sex among men with multiple partners. However, most school-based prevention focuses on heterosexual transmission, and while this can be effective in countries with generalized and hyperendemic scenarios, it does not address the three behaviors that put most Asian adolescents at risk. This highlights the importance for national AIDS authorities to "know their epidemic" if they are to implement successful responses. UNESCO believes that if schools were able to meet the educational needs of adolescents who engage in risky behaviors well before these adolescents engage in such behaviors, the impact of school-based HIV prevention programs on the course of Asian HIV/AIDS epidemics would be dramatically increased (De Lind van Wijngaarden et al., 2008).

This view is echoed in the 2009 report *Children and AIDS. Fourth Stocktaking Report* published by UNICEF in partnership with UNAIDS, WHO, and UNFPA. This annual report examines data on progress, emerging evidence, case studies of best practices and current knowledge, and practice for children as they relate to program areas known as the Four Ps: 1) preventing mother-to-child transmission of HIV; 2) providing pediatric HIV care and treatment; 3) preventing HIV infection among adolescents and young people; and 4) protecting and supporting children.

> The report finds that young men who have sex with men, young transgender people, young people involved in selling sex and young people injecting drugs are among the populations with the highest rates of HIV, yet few HIV programmes reach them. The evidence consistently shows that programmatic approaches focusing on pragmatic outcomes, such as reducing harm, are more effective than moralizing. Responses need to ensure that youth services and programmes respect the diversity of young people and respond to their needs, while recognizing the circumstances of most-at-risk groups and extending special protection to young people among them. (UNICEF, 2009, p. 34)

Prevention programs and more general responses that do not take into account local epidemic scenarios and do not address local behaviors will leave huge numbers of children and young people without the appropriate knowledge and skills to protect themselves. It is now widely acknowledged that there is no single global HIV epidemic, but that a range of epidemic scenarios may exist within a country or a region. This means that what works in South Africa will not necessarily work in India. To address this, UNAIDS developed a set of guidelines, entitled *Practical Guidelines for Intensifying HIV Prevention: Towards Universal Access*, that aims to encourage national AIDS authorities to "know their epidemic," that is, to recognize and understand what drives and characterizes the epidemic in their own country. Knowing their epidemic provides the basis for countries to "know their response" and helps them assess the extent to which their existing responses are meeting the needs of those most vulnerable to HIV infection.

Supportive learning environments

The international community is increasingly gearing its response toward universal access to prevention programs, treatment, care, and support, and the ways in which education systems and institutions can effectively contribute to this as well as other international development goals. This includes overcoming the underlying conditions that facilitate the spread of HIV such as poverty, ill health, gender inequality, and violence, particularly against girls and young women. Many believe that an educational institution's response to HIV/AIDS should be limited to HIV prevention. However, schools and other institutions are increasingly playing a significant role in supporting all the dimensions of a comprehensive response to HIV and AIDS including prevention, treatment, care, and support (UNESCO, 2008a).

Although school-based treatment, care, and support programs vary, UNESCO has identified a range of essential components that should be in place to provide a comprehensive response. For example, ensuring that children enroll and remain in school is crucial, not only so that they receive basic education but also so that students in need can access a range of support mechanisms in a caring and trusted environment. This can involve waiving school fees, introducing school feeding programs, providing support in the form of uniforms and school supplies, or making lessons more flexible for students who have to work or care for relatives. For example, a study conducted in Ethiopia found that schools that began and ended the school day earlier and scheduled breaks during the harvest period resulted in better pupil performance and retention (Verwimp, 1999).

In terms of treatment, educational institutions can help students and educators follow their treatment regime and raise awareness of how the side effects of antiretroviral therapy (ART) can affect teaching and learning outcomes. However, treatment education must be integrated across the continuum of HIV and AIDS education. Treatment education should not be seen as a separate component or an additional burden to already overstretched education and health systems but as an integral part of comprehensive HIV *and* AIDS education and should be included as part of planning processes to move toward universal access to prevention, treatment, care, and support (UNESCO and WHO, 2005).

Schools can also play an important role in providing psychosocial support either by training existing counselors to understand the impact of HIV and AIDS on students or by referring them to social services or nongovernmental organizations involved in this type of work. However, before this can take place, students infected or affected by HIV/AIDS need to be identified. Teachers and other staff can be trained to respond to the warning signs such as noticing if a student's appearance is worsening or schoolwork is deteriorating, and by keeping and analyzing records on absenteeism, lateness, and so on.

This, however, does not address the needs of the many children who have either never attended school or have dropped out. Incidentally, girls tend to be less likely to attend school due to a number of factors such as domestic duties, pregnancy, early marriage, the low value placed on girls' education, lack of household funds and unsafe learning environments. To reach these children, a range of different approaches has been identified, including accelerated educational programs for working children, teaching in places where children live and work, and making educational content, such as vocational training, more relevant.

Supporting teachers and educators

Most HIV/AIDS education responses tend to focus on learners and curricula and limited attention has been given to teachers and educators who often struggle to deal with challenges arising from the epidemic. Effective education sector responses depend on teacher education (both preservice and in-service) and support, and on educator commitment, confidence, knowledge, attitude, and skills (UNESCO, 2008b). Teachers are often ill-equipped to deliver prevention programs due to inadequate training and materials. Furthermore, talking about sex makes most teachers uncomfortable, and the same applies to inspectors, managers, and decision-makers who should be supporting teachers in their work. There are also varying amounts of "sexual policing" and what goes in the curriculum is often a compromise as a result of a highly political discussion (Clarke, 2008).

Recent data from a study on HIV-related knowledge uptake by sixth grade pupils in the 15 South African Development Community (SADC) countries revealed that, overall, 60 percent of the children in the most affected countries do not have a baseline knowledge of HIV/AIDS commensurate with the stated curricula. In comparison, it found that teachers generally *did* have a satisfactory minimum level of knowledge but that they were not passing on this knowledge to their students. It would be reasonable to suggest that this failure to transfer knowledge is attributable to the lack of proper training (SACMEQ, 2010).

An important initiative supportive of teachers is the EFAIDS teacher training program, launched in 2006, which is a partnership between Education International (EI), the World Health Organization (WHO) and EDC (Education Development Center). It is implemented by 46 teachers' unions in 35 countries. The program's aims are threefold: to prevent new HIV infections in teachers and learners; to mitigate the negative effects of AIDS on achieving the EFA goals; and to increase the number of learners completing basic education. The first goal is pursued via the training of teachers using exercises from *Teachers' Exercise Book on HIV Prevention.* The training is then passed on to other teachers and learners via a cascade system. The second goal is pursued by nurturing an open environment where risk reduction, testing, treatment, and care can be discussed and addressed. Achieving this goal entails conducting research on a variety of areas such as advocacy for the proper training, support, treatment, and care of teachers. Finally, the third goal is pursued via research, advocacy, and increasing public awareness. Between 2001 and 2005, the program had trained over 150,000 teachers in over 20,000 schools in 17 countries. An evaluation of the program reported a significant increase in teachers' knowledge of HIV prevention, teachers' acquisition of skill in using participatory learning exercises to train peers and students, teachers' guidance to students in obtaining further support and assistance, and the active role that motivation plays in HIV prevention (Pevzner, 2005).

On World AIDS Day 2007, EFAIDS launched the One Hour on AIDS initiative, which invites teachers and students around the world to spend one hour on AIDS. The lesson plan proposed in the activity kit helps participants to explore their knowledge and encourages them to express their views. Again, the cascade system is used and the lesson is taught in schools and union offices around the world, reinforcing the key role that teachers play in raising awareness of HIV/AIDS.

Another way in which educators and learners can be supported is through the implementation of education sector workplace policies. In 2004, the

International Labor Organization (ILO) launched a program to develop HIV/AIDS workplace policies for the education sector to complement the ILO Code of Practice on HIV/AIDS in the World of Work, which was adopted in 2001. In 2005, UNESCO collaborated with the ILO to develop an HIV/AIDS workplace policy to be used by education staff and stakeholders at both national and institutional levels. The policy covers six key areas: 1) prevention of HIV through workplace prevention; 2) education and training programs; 3) reduction of vulnerability arising from unequal gender and staff/student relationships; 4) elimination of stigma and discrimination on the basis of real or perceived HIV status and adherence to the rights of infected or affected staff and students; 5) care, treatment, and support of staff and students who are infected and/or affected by HIV/AIDS and management and mitigation of the impact of HIV/AIDS in education institutions; and 6) safe, healthy, and nonviolent work and study environments. This project has now been implemented in the Caribbean and Southern Africa, and UNESCO and ILO plan to expand the scope of the initiative to other regions.

In 2006, UNESCO together with the EI-EFAIDS program and WHO organized a consultation with HIV-positive teachers that brought together ministries of education (MoEs), teachers' unions and HIV-positive teachers' networks from six East and Southern African countries. The objectives of the consultation were to identify elements of comprehensive responses for HIV-positive teachers based on experience and lessons learned in Kenya, Namibia, Tanzania, Uganda, Zambia, and Zimbabwe. Given the sensitive nature of the issue, many MoEs and trade unions are uncertain about how to respond to the needs of HIV-positive teachers and even though many workplace policies have been developed, few specifically address the needs of teachers, or indeed students, living with HIV.

One of the most urgent issues for teachers was to be able to access affordable and confidential health, treatment, care, and support services. Many teachers at the conference who were receiving ART explained that without support from the school, managing their treatment could be problematic. Regular visits to hospitals (sometimes up to two days away) meant taking time off work, which in turn increased their colleagues' workload. Teachers were also worried that frequent absences from school could arouse suspicion among colleagues, students, and parents if they had not disclosed their status. The participants in the consultation recommended that links be made with existing public treatment structures and that partnerships be created rather than setting up specific programs for teachers, which could unintentionally increase stigmatization.

Funding

AIDS-related funding from the international community for low- and middle-income countries comes from three main funding streams: donations from national governments, multilateral funding organizations, and private funding. From the 1990s until 2009, funding for the AIDS epidemic increased substantially. In 2008, an estimated US$15.6 billion was spent on HIV/AIDS compared to US$300 million in 1996 (UNAIDS, 2006, 2008). From 2002 to 2008, funding increased sixfold. However, since 2009, total global funding for HIV/AIDS has remained flat. Furthermore, there are growing concerns about a reduction in nonhealth-sector funding for HIV/AIDS. Most funding for HIV/AIDS is now provided by the Global Fund for AIDS, Tuberculosis and Malaria (GFATM) and the US President's Emergency Plan for AIDS Relief (PEPFAR), both of which tend to direct their funds through ministries of health, and while some of these funds do trickle down to the education sector, it is not a major recipient of these funds per se. Furthermore, the Department for International Development (DFID), one of the world's biggest bilateral donors for HIV/AIDS, announced in 2008 that its emphasis would be on strengthening health systems rather than on HIV/AIDS specifically. DFID is also a major donor to the GFATM.

Other funding for HIV/AIDS is provided by the Education for All Fast Track Initiative (EFA FTI), which is a global partnership between donor and developing countries to ensure accelerated progress toward the MDG of universal primary education by 2015. All low-income countries that demonstrate a serious commitment to achieving this goal can join the FTI. For their part, developing countries commit to developing and implementing credible and sustainable education plans that must also include a strategy for addressing HIV/AIDS, gender equality, and other key issues, and to increasing domestic finance for primary education. In turn, donor countries, multilateral organizations, and civil-society organizations commit to align their support to these education sector plans through increased cooperation, harmonization, and financial support. However, in order to receive funding, countries must first have their education plans appraised and then endorsed by the FTI. In 2008, a working group of the IATT, in collaboration with the EFA FTI, carried out an assessment in eight countries of the responsiveness to HIV/AIDS of education sector plans that were endorsed by the FTI between 2004 and 2006. The report found that three of the countries' plans had been endorsed without any HIV/AIDS components at all and two countries' plans had been endorsed with only a limited set of HIV-related interventions (Bundy et al., 2008).

Conclusion

This review of the education sector's response to HIV/AIDS is by no means exhaustive, but it is hoped that it illustrates how, through coordinated, multisectoral efforts, progress is being made in both mitigating the impact of the epidemic on education systems and providing learners and educators with the knowledge, values, and skills required to protect themselves and others. While much has been achieved, especially in terms of accessing antiretroviral therapy and delivering prevention programs, much more remains to be done if this progress is to be sustained and scaled up.

Gains have been made through the health sector, but there has been less progress in mainstreaming HIV/AIDS in other sectors. Although few would dispute that strong health systems are essential to effective HIV/AIDS responses, evidence demonstrates that a multisectoral approach with the education sector playing a key role can leverage a much wider variety of resources in order to produce better health outcomes. Programs must be taken out of isolation; positioning the response to HIV/AIDS within the broader development agenda will accelerate progress toward all the MDGs and optimize increasingly scarce resources. However, domestic budgetary constraints, declining levels of aid, and the ongoing impact of the financial crisis will put many developing nations in serious danger of rolling back the gains already made to expand access to education. Recent analysis indicates that if current trends continue, there will be more children out of school in 2015 than there are today (UNESCO, 2009). It is essential that ongoing and serious investment in education is seen as an integral part of the response to HIV and AIDS and to achieving broader development goals.

Questions for reflection

1. In what ways does the "educational response" aim at impacting the HIV/AIDS epidemic?
2. What are some common limitations to the "educational response?"
3. How is the institution of education commonly impacted by HIV/AIDS?

Acknowledgements

The authors would like to acknowledge the contribution of Lucy Teasdale (consultant) to the preparation of this chapter.

Reference list

ActionAid International and Save the Children Fund, UK (2004). *HIV/AIDS and Education, Life-skills-based Education for hiv Prevention: a Critical Analysis.* London: UK Working Group on Education and HIV & AIDS.

Bundy, D., A. Patrikios, C. Mannathoko, A. Tembon, S. Manda. B. Sarr, and L. Drake. (2007). *Accelerating the Education Sector Response to HIV and AIDS: Five Years On.* Washington, DC: The International Bank for Reconstruction and Development and the World Bank.

Bundy, D., and D. J. Clarke (2008). *The EFA Fast Track Initiative: An Assessment of the Responsiveness of Endorsed Education Sector Plans to HIV and AIDS.* Paris: Interagency Task Team (IATT) on Education.

Clarke, D. J. (2008). *Heroes and Villains: Teachers in the Education Response to hiv.* Paris: UNESCO/IIEP.

Commission on AIDS in Asia (2008). *Redefining AIDS in Asia: Crafting an Effective Response.* New Delhi: Oxford University Press.

De Lind van Wijngaarden, J., and S. Shaeffer (2008). *UNESCO's Response to the Report of the Commission of AIDS in Asia.* Bangkok: UNESCO.

Gallant, M., and E. Maticka-Tyndale (2004). "School-based HIV prevention programmes for African youth." *Social Science and Medicine* 58, 1337–51.

Hargreaves, J. R., and T. Boler (2006). *Girl Power: The Impact of Girls' Education on hiv and Sexual Behaviour.* London: ActionAid International.

Hargreaves, J. R., C. P. Bonell, T. Boler, D. Boccia, I. Birdthistle, A. Fletcher, P. M. Pronyk, and J. R. Glyn. (2008). 'Systematic review exploring time trends in the association between educational attainment and risk of HIV infection in sub-Saharan Africa.' *AIDS*, 22, 403–14.

Kelly, M. J. (2000). *Planning for Education in the Context of HIV/AIDS.* Paris: UNESCO IIEP.

Kirby, D. (2007). *Emerging Answers 2007: Research Findings on Programs to Reduce Teen Pregnancy and Sexually Transmitted Diseases.* Washington, DC: The National Campaign to Prevent Teen and Unplanned Pregnancy.

Pevzner, E. (2005). *A Report on the World Health Organization (WHO), Education International (EI), and Education Development Center's (EDC) Teacher Training Program to Prevent hiv Infection and Related Discrimination.* Chapel Hill: University of North Carolina.

SACMEQ (2010). "How successful are HIV-AIDS prevention education programs?" *Policy Issues Series* 8, September.

UNAIDS (2006). *Report on the Global AIDS Epidemic.* Geneva: UNAIDS.

— (2008). *Report on the Global AIDS Epidemic.* Geneva: UNAIDS.

— (2009). *AIDS Epidemic Update*. Geneva: UNAIDS and WHO.

UNESCO (2006). *Linking educaids with Other On-Going Initiatives: An Overview of Opportunities: An Assessment of Challenges*. Paris: UNESCO.

— (2008a). *Educator Development and Support, Good Policy and Practice in HIV & AIDS and Education*. Booklet 3, Booklet Series. Paris: UNESCO.

— (2008b). *School-Centred HIV and AIDS Care and Support in Southern Africa: Technical Consultation Report, 22–24 May 2008, Gaborone, Botswana*. Paris: UNESCO.

— (2009). *EDUCAIDS Evaluation 2009: Key Findings, Recommendations and UNESCO's Actions*. Paris: UNESCO.

UNESCO and WHO (2005). *HIV and AIDS. Treatment Education: Technical Consultation Report, 22 November to 23 November 2005, Paris, France*. Paris: UNESCO and WHO.

UNICEF, UNAIDS, WHO, UNFPA and UNESCO (2009). *Children and AIDS: Fifth Stocktaking Report*. New York: UNICEF, UNAIDS, WHO, UNFPA, and UNESCO.

United Nations (2010). *The Millennium Development Goals Report 2010*. New York: United Nations.

Verwimp, P. (1999). "Measuring the quality of education at two levels: a case study of primary schools in rural Ethiopia." *International Review of Education* 5 (2), 167–96.

World Bank (2002). *Education and HIV/AIDS: A Window of Hope*. Washington, DC: World Bank.

The Politics of the President's Emergency Plan for AIDS Relief (PEPFAR)

David Kovara

2

Introduction

In May 2003, President George W. Bush signed H.R. 1298, the Global AIDS Bill, authorizing $15 billion for HIV/AIDS interventions around the world. Passing through the US Congress in less than three months, this bill provided the legal framework for a policy document released nearly one year later and now known as the President's Emergency Plan for AIDS Relief (PEPFAR, or the Emergency Plan), in which the Bush administration detailed a five-year strategy to "turn the tide" of the global HIV/AIDS pandemic. The body of this chapter was written during the presidency of George W. Bush. Since the inauguration of President Barack Obama, much has changed. The histories and analyses presented in this chapter, however, are still useful in understanding the political nature of HIV/AIDS education.

This chapter discusses two of the more controversial provisions and compromises evident in PEPFAR:

1. A requirement that 33 percent of PEPFAR's prevention budget, or roughly 7 percent of the overall budget, be reserved for "abstinence-until-marriage" programs, referred to in this chapter as ABY.
2. A "conscience clause" ensuring that faith-based organizations (FBOs) will still be fully eligible for prevention funding even if they refuse to promote messages (such as condom use) that may conflict with their articles of faith.

Both of these provisions were the result of intensive lobbying by evangelical Christian-interest groups based in Washington, DC, at least six of which were determined to align the Global AIDS Bill with the values of social conservatives. Both provisions would, in practice, advance the stated preference of the Bush administration to partner more extensively with faith-based organizations (FBOs) around the world. Indeed, after PEPFAR's legislation, the lion's share of abstinence funding would be awarded to local and international FBOs, many of whom were founded upon explicit missionary mandates: an evangelical Christian imperative to target local communities, even entire nations, for conversion to Christianity.

The goal of this chapter is to analyze the lobbying activities and rhetoric of six special-interest groups, representing the socially conservative platform of evangelical Christians in the United States of America during the Congressional legislation of the Global AIDS Bill. With frequent reference to the literature on "morality politics" and "interest-group politics," this chapter will explain how these groups used a sophisticated "inside-outside" strategy to directly effect seven targeted changes to the Global AIDS Bill, including the creation of both its abstinence-until-marriage earmark and conscience clause for FBOs.

Morality policy and politics

"Morality politics" is a phrase used to describe debates where at least "one advocacy coalition" portrays an issue "in terms of morality or sin and use[ing] moral arguments in its policy advocacy" (Haider-Markel et al., 1996, p. 333). The goal of this advocacy is to obtain government validation, or "authoritative legitimization" of one set of values or rights over another (Vergari, 2001, p. 201).

Arguments over abortion policy are a typical example of morality politics because they use uncompromising moral positions regarding the definition of life, of personhood, of a female's right to control her body, and of the limits of government in the sphere of our private lives. However, as Mooney (2001, p. 4) points out, not all "moral" issues will necessarily result in morality politics, just as some seemingly technical issues such as carbon emissions can with the right rhetoric take on deeply controversial moral significance. Politics and policies take on a moral nature based on the way the debate is framed and the perspectives and perceptions of the actors involved. "If at least one advocacy coalition involved in the debate defines the issue as threatening one of its core values," Mooney explains, "we have a morality policy."

There are two specific elements of these debates that are important to understand the impact of morality politics on HIV/AIDS education. First, morality politics actors tend to "overstate the need for governmental response" (Blankenau and Leeper, 2003, p. 567). The subjects of morality policy evoke heightened passions and rhetoric, leading to unusually urgent statements about the need for formal regulation.

Second, as Goggin and Mooney (2001, p. 138) note, in these debates lawmakers tend "not to solicit information as often, to rely more on information based on the personal experiences of their informants and others, and to listen and to learn from this information only selectively." In addition to the use of selective information, these lawmakers tend to engage in expressive (as opposed to instrumental) debates and processes. The questions addressed by policymakers are not about "what works" according to evidence, but rather about the validation of specific values and principles.

While researchers have explored these issues in terms of the relationship between Christian values and US politics as well as the battlefront of "abstinence-only" sex education, the case of PEPFAR represents a distinct departure from this literature in several ways.

First, PEPFAR is a US foreign policy intended for use in Africa. Most research on morality politics, as of 2010, has focused mainly on domestic US politics. Second, the specific use of PEPFAR as HIV/AIDS prevention shifts the topic slightly outside previous scholarship on abstinence education disputes. Third, the politics surrounding PEPFAR involve significant participation by special-interest groups, as the next section explains.

Morality politics and special-interest groups

There are two contradictory perspectives on the actions of special-interest groups. The first position holds that the role of interest groups in policy formation is diminishing; increased access to information has decreased politicians' reliance on these groups to inform them on specific issues. Furthermore, interest groups tend to function most effectively behind the scenes when the larger public is apathetic. In the case of morality politics, which are to some extent defined by public engagement and interest, lawmakers are more responsive to perceived citizen preferences than to the interests of a smaller lobby (Norrander and Wilcox, 2001).

The contrasting perspective argues that special-interest groups play a significant role in shaping morality politics, by "framing the issue" in ways that appeal to lawmakers, keeping public salience low, and by providing "resources" such as campaign donations, volunteers, and electoral support (Haider-Markel, 2001; Pierce and Miller, 2001). Crucially, if interest groups can "demoralize" the issue and thus keep public interest low, their influence on the political process appears to increase.

Of course, religious lobbyists are not a new phenomenon. The organized activity of evangelical lobbyists in Washington, DC has been documented as early as the late 1970s and into the 1980s, (Fowler et al., 1999; Hertzke, 1988; Neuhaus et al., 1987); this activity was enabled at the time by the ideologies of born-again Christianity and by the political ideologies of Carter and, more importantly, Ronald Reagan (Hutcheson, 1989). As Loomis and Cigler note on contemporary politics, "Christian right mobilization has been widely credited for reenergizing the Republican Party, helping it gain control of both houses of Congress in 1994 and the presidency in 2000" (introduction to Guth et al., 2007). To put it even more directly: under G. W. Bush and his Republican Congresses, it is possible evangelical interest groups have achieved higher levels of political access and influence—and their allies, more key administrative posts—than ever before.

Context

When the Global AIDS Bill was initially taken up by Congress in March 2003, it was a bipartisan document drafted by Congressman Hyde (a conservative) and

Congressman Lantos (a liberal) with concessions made on both sides of the aisle. To Washington conservatives, however, the bill was unacceptable, and just a few days after its release, a list outlining the "Conservative Top Ten Goals for Global AIDS Bill" was drafted and circulated. Using these ten goals as a reference point, it is useful to compare the initial Global AIDS Bill with its final version.

Seven conservative provisions found their way into the legislation in less than two months. And since two provisions were already present in the original bill, it appears that only one conservative goal—concerning abortion—failed to be realized, a victory that did not go unnoticed by lobbyists: "When the US Senate passed the Global AIDS bill on last Thursday, May 8, it came as a victory for conservatives, who succeeded in getting seven out of ten of their provisions included in what had become a controversial piece of legislation" (CWA, May 19, 2003).

Indeed after the bill's public release, religious interest groups were quick to take credit for its conservative provisions. "I am confident," said Ken Connor, president of the Family Research Council, "that were it not for the leadership of groups like FRC, Focus on the Family, Prison Fellowship, and, in particular, FRC's Government Affairs division, led by Vice President Connie Mackey, the AIDS bill the Senate passed last month would have been a complete disaster. Our groups worked tirelessly over the past three months to fix a bad bill and ensure that the final legislation reflected sound pro-family principles" (Figart, 2003).

These claims of success, however, are not intrinsically convincing. It would be unusual for a lobby group in Washington not to claim responsibility for legislative victories: funding, membership, and staff morale depend upon maintaining an image of influence, however dubious. In order to understand whether and how Christian lobby groups succeeded in altering the Global AIDS Bill, it is necessary to go beyond public claims of success and instead search for evidence regarding what possible effect a lobbying body might have on lawmakers.

Methods

The policy research grounding this chapter began with 16 key informant interviews at USAID, the Government Accountability Office, Congressional offices, one academic researcher, and representatives from Washington, DC-based nonprofits. Significant document analysis was also completed, focusing on Congressional records and the publications of special-interest groups.

The legal basis for PEPFAR is found in "The US Leadership against Malaria, HIV/AIDS and Tuberculosis Act of 2003," more colloquially known as the Global AIDS Bill (USGov, 2003). Congress had four opportunities to shape the legal basis for PEPFAR and one opportunity to alter its financial framework.

By the time President Bush signed the Global AIDS Bill into law, Congress had publicly debated 37 different amendments. Transcripts from these debates and statements were isolated if they were in any way related to:

1. the abstinence earmark tabled by Rep. Joe Pitts (R-Pa), first in committee, then in the House;
2. the "conscience clause" amendment, also tabled twice: first by Pitts in Committee, second by Rep. Chris Smith (R-NJ) in the House.

Each statement or section of debate related to either of these issues was analyzed for recurring themes and arguments. The words were also counted to determine a very rough approximation of how much Congressional energy was spent debating abstinence promotion.

The next stage of analysis applied themes found in morality policy research—for example, whether positions overstated the need for government involvement—which were compared to the rhetoric of lobbying agencies, generating insights about synergy between Congressional positions and special-interest groups.

To determine which groups were active in the politics of the bill, profiles were reviewed of 61 "right-wing" organizations identified by People for the American Way as politically active. Eventually it became clear that six evangelical Christian interest groups were active in the politics of the Global AIDS Bill. After searching all available materials related to their activities on the abstinence amendment in the Global AIDS Bill, approximately 30 publications were found, roughly one publication per week during the legislative period.

Findings: The actors

The lobbyists

At least six conservative special-interest groups shaped the politics of the Global AIDS Bill:

1. Family Research Council (FRC)
2. Focus on the Family (FoF)

3. BreakPoint/Prison Fellowships (BP)
4. Concerned Women for America/Beverley LaHaye Institute (CWA)
5. Eagle Forum (EF)
6. Traditional Values Coalition (TVC)

These six interest groups are related to each other in a number of ways. The FRC, for example, was originally founded by James Dobson to be the "political arm" of FoF (Crowley, 2004). The FRC, FoF, TVC, and CWA have been credited with the successful, harmonized mobilization of values voters in 2004, a crucial voting bloc in G. W. Bush's re-election (Guth et al., 2007, p. 158). A review of their mission statements shows that five of the six groups operate under similar, explicitly evangelical mandates, promoting biblical values in both private and public spheres as a moral imperative.

In additional to their shared evangelical mandates and lineage, these six groups are also related in a Congressional context: that is, at least five of them are members of the Values Action Teams in both the House and Senate. Although very little is on record about the VAT, the following section will provide what background there is.

The Values Action Team

In 1998, around the time of the annual values summit in Washington, James Dobson, head of the Focus on the Family media empire and one of America's most recognizable—and possibly most influential (Gilgoff, 2007)—evangelical Christian personalities of the past 20 years, threatened to leave the Republican Party for neglecting what he considered key moral issues: "I want them to listen to the people who put them in power," said Dobson. "I want them to pay attention to the issues that burn within the hearts of the primary constituency of the Republican Party [. . .] If they won't do that, then they ought to lose" (Schuman, 1998).

Afraid to lose Dobson and his affiliates, the Republicans offered to create a Values Action Team—or VAT—in the House of Representatives: an "off-the-record" caucus, housed in the Republican Study Committee, linking members of the House of Representatives to conservative Christian lobby groups (Blumenthal, 2009). Tom DeLay and Michael Schwartz supervised its establishment, opening "an official and permanent communications channel," as Gilgoff (2007, p. 115) puts it, "between dozens of Religious Right groups and Republican lawmakers," creating, for the first time, a forum "allowing socially conservative congressmen to leverage the huge mailing lists of out-side groups like the Family Research Council in lobbying wavering fellow members on key votes."

Since its inception, the House VAT has met every Thursday after-noon, bringing together roughly 30 interest groups with staff from 70 Congressional offices. From the beginning it has been chaired by Joseph Pitts (R-Pa). And due to its popularity in the House, a sister VAT was established in the Senate in 2002, chaired by Sam Brownback. Neither the House nor Senate VAT is merely a fellowship gathering: they are serious, weekly strategic sessions in which legislation is discussed and tasks are divided among the members. "I'll say [to the outside groups], 'Who will do letters?' 'Who will do radio shows?' 'Who will contact these members?' and we strategize about tactics," Pitts is quoted as saying (Gilgoff, 2007, p. 115). "Working together we can be much more effective. In politics, it's not always the wisest or the strongest who wins, it's the most persist-ent. The [outside groups] have to stay at it long-term, and never, never go away. And if they work together and are persistent, they can advance their priorities."

Specific membership lists for both the House and Senate VATS are diffi-cult to locate. Gilgoff (2007) suggests there were a dozen Republican members when it started in 1998, and that by 2006, there were about 70, "accounting for roughly one in every six members of Congress" (p. 132). Concrete numbers are hard to find, in part because of the secrecy surrounding the group's activ-ities. A VAT membership list used to be posted on Joseph Pitts's website, but by April 2007, it had been password protected, and by June 2008, the page was removed entirely. All links to the VAT on the Republican Study Committee website were down by April 2007. As Sharlet (2006) writes in a profile of Sam Brownback:

> Everything that is said is strictly off the record, and even the groups themselves are forbidden from discussing the proceedings. It's a little "cloak-and-dagger," says a Brownback press secretary. The VAT is a war council, and the enemy, says one participant, is "secularism."

Conclusively linking the VAT to the conservative provisions of PEPFAR may not be possible, but it would explain how Christian lobbyists—at least in the case of the Global AIDS Bill—waged such an organized and responsive campaign.

Findings: The strategies of conservative special-interest groups

Overview

In order to align the Global AIDS Bill with conservative Christian values, special-interest groups deployed a sophisticated "inside-outside" lobbying strategy. On the "inside," lobbyists collaborated with Congressional staffers through weekly VAT meetings, developing amendments such as the abstinence earmark as well as crafting arguments and scripts for use during floor debates. On the "outside," lobbyists engaged in extensive citizen mobilization, prompting their membership base to exert pressure on the legislative process. This inside-outside strategy, which may also be described as a combination of direct and indirect lobbying, is illustrated in Figure 1 below:

Narrative of time line

The Global AIDS Bill, a bipartisan document, was introduced by Hyde and Lantos on March 17, 2003. One day later, the conservative lobby began publishing articles and "action alerts," brief, policy-oriented messages sent by

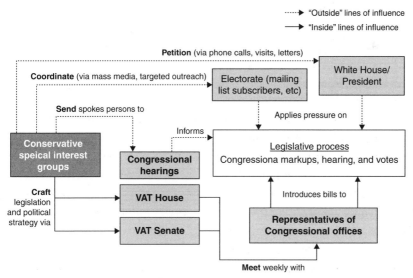

Figure 1 "Inside-Outside" strategy of conservative lobbying groups

e-mail to a considerably large list of subscribers. Specifically, before the committee had even met to discuss the first draft bill, FoF had criticized it with one publication and CWA with two: among other deficiencies in the bill, they argued, abstinence "takes a back seat" to condoms and faith-based organizations are not protected by a conscience clause (CWA, March 31, 2003; Fof, March 18, 2003).

When the committee met on April 2 to mark up the draft legislation, Joseph Pitts (chair of the House Values Action Team) became the champion of both concerns, introducing an amendment "prioritizing" abstinence promotion, as well as a conscience clause for protecting faith-based organizations. Both amendments failed, voted down by a Democratic majority. And so over the next two weeks, interest groups released a flurry of action alerts and radio broadcasts to their subscribers. CWA, for example, labeled the bill reprehensible, "on a downward spiral," and called for it to be replaced with something "clean" that "actually saves lives" (CWA, April 9, 2003).

Importantly, many of these criticisms were accompanied by detailed instructions to listeners and readers on how to impact the Congressional debates. Phone numbers were listed, form letters were drafted, and even automatic e-mail generators were provided. Chuck Colson of BP exemplified the urgent rhetoric, suggesting to his readers this was:

> One of the most important bills that has been offered by our government. As the president said, it will define what kind of nation we are. I don't say this often, but we need you [. . .] Take action: Urge your congressman to support the amendments to the AIDS bill (H. R. 1298) that make abstinence first and provide a conscience clause for faith-based organizations. The Capitol switchboard is 1-202-224-3121 (BP, April 30, 2003).

In addition to sending out detailed action alerts, conservative lobbyists communicated with the White House. On April 29, for example, President Bush held private meetings with "about a dozen" religious leaders, in which they urged him to veto any bill that did not prioritize abstinence (Eckstrom, 2003). Detailed letters to the administration were also sent, such as a long statement from EF once again asking the president not to sign a bill that did not contain the necessary conservative provisions (EF, 2003a).

And yet, despite the concerns of conservatives—indeed, over their objections—President Bush still chose to champion the bill, holding a Rose Garden speech to articulate his support. Three days later, as the House convened to debate the Global AIDS Bill, Rep. Nadler (D-NY) praised the president for his apparent willingness to defy Christian lobbyists:

> I'm particularly pleased that President Bush has stood up to the extremists in his party who wished to hijack this bill to push their ideological agenda . . . When the Traditional Values Coalition and the Family Research Council are opposed to legislation, we must be doing something right. (CR May 1, 2003, p. H3588)

As it turned out, Nadler spoke too soon. As the EF had already predicted, Joe Pitts would indeed use the introduction of the bill to the entire House floor as an opportunity to reintroduce another abstinence amendment, while fellow conservative Christopher Smith (R-NJ) introduced a conscience-clause amendment. This time, both amendments were voted through, and the Conservative lobby achieved an unlikely victory: convincing the House to "send life, not death, to Africa" (CWA, May 1, 2003), in what Pitts called "an infinitely better Bill" (CWA, April 30, 2003).

At this point in the legislative process, however, lawmakers still appeared to believe that the abstinence amendment would never actually make it into law. As a senior legislative aide to Bill Frist explained to me in a telephone interview: "Nobody thought [abstinence] would be the answer . . . They thought, we're not agreeing to something final here; we'll keep the social conservatives happy, then fix it later. We'll have time, because that's how the process works" (Interview, October 6, 2006).

Thus the conservative lobby shifted tactics. Having won a victory in the House, they altered the rhetoric of their mailings by calling upon the Senate to pass the bill immediately, without changes (any changes would have sent the bill back to the House for "conference" in which differences would be negotiated).

Their rhetorical tactic was twofold: first, they insisted that every second spent debating was another second of people dying from AIDS: "Men, women and children are dying in Africa; this is no time for political games" a release from CWA read, "[. . .] In the battle against AIDS, every delay equals death" (CWA, May 15, 2003). Similarly worded releases came from FoF, including a letter sent to Bill Frist, signed by 13 religious-interest groups, urging him to pass the bill quickly. And Chuck Colson released his own commentary, warning that if we "lose Africa" to AIDS, radical Islam could take over (BP, May 14, 2003).

Second, they appeared to have recruited the White House into the lobbying campaign. "On May 2," explained Frist's legislative aide, "the House passes the bill. Within weeks, the White House was saying, we want this bill passed, so the president can take it to the G8 meeting, so the president can challenge the other heads of state" (Interview, October 6, 2006).

The tactics of the conservative lobby appeared to pay off. Bill Frist, senate majority leader, introduced the bill with a strongly worded exhortation to pass it without changes:

> We must pass this bill. We must pass this bill this week . . . It is a moral issue, and history will ultimately judge how this body responds to this devastating virus. There is no change I could personally propose to this legislation that is so signifi-cant that it would cause a delay in getting this bill to the President. (CR, May 13, 2003, p. S6037).

Under the leadership of Frist, the Republicans united and, wielding a major-ity vote, were able to defeat every amendment as it appeared, including one from Dianne Feinstein (D-Ca) to repeal the abstinence earmark, introduced at midnight. "The Republicans stayed united," confirms the aide, "and because of the partisan votes, the Republicans beat down these amendments" (Interview, October 6, 2006).

When the Senate finally passed the Global AIDS Bill (with one minor change), conservatives were once again able to issue rather exuberant announcements. "Everyone who contributed to this result," wrote Sandy Rios of CWA, "deserves the congratulations and the gratitude of the entire human race, for they have done something important for all of humanity." Indeed, because of the way abstinence and fidelity "cultivate" character, this bill "may prove to be one of the greatest events in the history of Africa" (CWA, May 16, 2003).

FoF likewise called the bill a "triumph for the abstinence movement," ask-ing its members to first "give thanks to God that the Congress has passed a bill for fighting AIDS that honors God's principles," and second, "thank President Bush and Senate Majority Leader Frist for their hard work [. . .] Thank them especially for acknowledging the importance of abstinence in preventing HIV/AIDS" (FoF, May 16, 2003).

There were still more policy battles to come. The legal framework had suc-cessfully passed but the fiscal framework, the money, was still up for debate. Within two weeks of the bill's passage, approximately 250 ministers, mission-aries, and donors converged on Washington to lobby for funds. Organized by World Vision (which would eventually secure a $10 million abstinence grant), the National Association of Evangelicals, and MAP International, the group was briefed by Karl Rove before dividing into groups to meet with about 20 lawmakers (Cooperman, 2003).

A period of relative quiet followed the evangelical conference. Congress would not take up the Global AIDS Bill again until October, when the Appropriations Act was set to be passed, authorizing funds for fiscal year 2004. Not surprisingly, the Appropriations Act was controversial. Several provisions had been passed somewhat surreptitiously in the House and Senate committees that were upsetting to the conservative lobby, including one provision that would assign most of the money to the jurisdiction of USAID and another that watered down the conscience-clause amendment. Equally alarming to the lobby was an amendment put forward by Sen. Feinstein: a recalibration of the prevention budget guidelines which would effectively reduce the 33-percent abstinence earmark.

FoF responded to these developments by issuing a detailed action alert two weeks before the deliberations, announcing to its members that the Global AIDS Bill was "in jeopardy" (FoF, Oct. 13, 2003). The alert included a "crash course" on Congressional procedure so that readers could follow the intricacies of the issue. In a separate action alert, released three days later and also entitled "Global AIDS Bill in Jeopardy," the TVC claimed that "what began as an honest effort to promote abstinence instead of condom distribution as a way of solving the AIDS crisis overseas, has been hijacked by the condom-giveaway advocates," otherwise known as "procondom, prohomosexual groups in government" (TVC, Oct. 16, 2003).

In additional to action alerts, lobbyists once again secured assistance from the executive branch, this time soliciting the Global AIDS Coordinator, Randall Tobias, to compose a letter to senators on the Foreign Appropriations Subcommittee opposing the Feinstein amendment. "The effect of this amendment," he wrote, "would be to decrease the amount that could be spent on abstinence-until-marriage programs as a prevention method, and I believe that would not be in the interest of best public health practice" (see TVC, Oct. 31, 2003).

On the day of the Senate consideration, the Feinstein amendment failed by a slim margin (45 to 47), and with additional amendments from Bill Frist, all of the Global AIDS Bill's original provisions were restored. So once again it was a nearly comprehensive victory for conservatives, and again the requisite congratulatory alerts were sent out, including one from FoF crediting not only Tobias but also, interestingly, voter pressure: "In addition to Tobias' letter," Izsak said, "phone calls, faxes and e-mails from Americans urging their senators to support Bush's plan for international AIDS prevention were crucial to the outcome of the vote." And that's just the way it's supposed to be, according to Bill Wichterman, policy adviser to Senate Majority Leader Bill Frist, R-Tn. "This is how democracy works," Wichterman told CitizenLink. "I'm not cynical about the process. This is still a place where constituents lead" (FoF, Oct. 31, 2003).

In this section I have shown a temporal relationship between lobbying and Congressional actions, and I believe this narrative of events offers persuasive evidence for the impact of Christian lobbyists.

Findings: The rhetoric

Conservative lobbyists and functional rhetoric

The abstinence earmark pushed by conservative lobbyists was clearly linked to their Christian beliefs: their position, in other words, was grounded in the "first principles" of conservative sexual morality. "Acting now," wrote Chuck Colson of BP, "is a moral imperative. But morally concerned citizens must also fight hard to make sure that America does not inadvertently give money to international groups that focus on condom distribution—or that promote abortion. I have the president's assistants' personal assurance that the administration will not do this" (BP, March 17, 2003).

In their publications, however, special-interest groups appeared to have largely avoided first-principle arguments. For example, a word search of all 30 publications issued by Christian lobbyists for the words *sin*, *evil*, *bad*, *wrong*, *right*, *good*, *values*, *bible*, *biblical*, *scriptural*, and *God*, returned only three examples. Instead the vast majority of publications argued for abstinence promotion with thinly functional terms (rather than thickly moral ones), namely that abstinence promotion "works," in contrast to "failed" condom promotion policies of the past. Of the 30 special-interest publications, for example, 22 cited the example of Uganda and its ABC strategy—"a model," the EF explained with typical inaccuracy, that "prioritizes abstinence, being faithful to a monogamous partner, and only as a last resort, condoms," (EF, 2003b).

To be clear, however, no policy brief or action alert devoted more than one paragraph to the Uganda example, and no publication offered more than two passing references to academic literature (typically authored by one researcher, Edward Green). Thus, although emphasis on the Ugandan model was apparently meant to serve a functional rather than "expressive" purpose in the lobbying materials, such efforts could by no means be classified as evidence of "technical" or "complex" arguments in the same way that environmental groups, for example, may provide detailed reports on carbon emissions. The ABC model of Uganda was in this case a thin functional argument covering an underlying moral agenda, but it was enough to allow lobbyists to claim they were pushing for "science-based" amendments. Ultimately this tactic may have been enough to "de-moralize" the issue, in effect restricting public salience to their own membership lists.

Congress and functional rhetoric

Only a few Republicans argued for abstinence promotion on clearly moral grounds. "It strikes me," Pence (R-In) announced, "as I rise to support the Pitts [abstinence] amendment and oppose the secondary amendment by Ms. Lee, that as we undertake a moral imperative, Mr. Chairman, I think it is important that we do it morally and we do it in a way that in some way reflects the moral character of the people of the United States of America" (IR, April 2, 2003).

Instead, like the lobbyists, the vast majority of Republicans argued for abstinence with thinly functional references to Uganda's success and the ABC model, though, again, the Congressional estimations of Uganda's success were vague, oversimplified, and at times distorted. Weldon (R-Fl), for example, suggested that "Uganda had faith. Uganda had faith in God and in its people to save themselves. President Museveni asked his people to change their behavior in order to stay alive," (CR, May 21, 2003, p. H4377). In a similar vein, the so-called ABC model was invoked repeatedly as an explanation for Uganda's success, though ABC was presented as different things by different members of Congress, sometimes in the same sentence. Ryan (R-Ks), for example, seemed to believe that ABC was either a "program" or a "model of behavior," but did not specify which. "[Uganda's success] has been accomplished through the ABC program, a model of behavior that we need to follow. First of all, abstinence; second, be faithful; and, third, using a condom" (CR, May 1, 2003, p. H3614).

Such statements indicated an abiding Congressional confusion over what ABC actually is. Indeed, in general, the Congressional debate demonstrates an apparent failure to engage with, or perhaps deliberate disregard for, the growing body of research regarding successful HIV prevention campaigns. Perhaps as a result, the practical ramifications of an abstinence earmark were almost completely ignored in the debate. Indeed, only three democrats bothered to question what people were actually talking about, including Senator Lantos (D-Ca) who tried to figure out what the Pitts amendment would mean in practice:

> Does the Pitts amendment seek to replicate certain abstinence-only programs under which educators are explicitly prohibited from giving full and complete information about condoms to high-risk populations? Under these abstinence set-aside programs, will people who are already sexually active be given any information about condoms? [. . .] And questions along these lines too numerous to mention. (CR, May 1, 2003, p. H3613).

He received no answers. (In rather backwards fashion, the Senate convened a hearing—entitled Fighting Aids in Uganda: What Went Right?—on May 19, three days after PEPFAR had already been legislated). Sen. Feinstein (D-Ca) also continued to look for answers: as late as October, during the appropriations process, she announced to the floor that she had sought a clear definition of abstinence-until-marriage by writing to Paul Kelly, Assistant Secretary of State for Legislative Affairs, and that his response, not surprisingly, made generic reference to ABC without offering concrete guidance or definitions of what would be funded.

Thus, with few exceptions, ABC appears to be invoked repeatedly yet vaguely as a "proven" formula upon which a global AIDS intervention should be modeled, suggesting that some members of Congress were merely repeating concepts that were recognizable in an ideological way without taking on board the research behind the concepts, or the implications of legislating them. The debates were in this regard expressive and not at all instrumental, a classic feature of morality policy in general.

Conservative lobbyists and rhetoric on government regulation

In addition to their thinly functional rhetoric, all six interest groups repeatedly claimed that without legislative amendments, the US government would continue to support failed HIV prevention policies around the world, wasting "billions of taxpayer dollars." They were, in the words of morality politics scholarship, "overstating the need for government regulation" (Blankenau and Leeper, 2003, p. 567). Specifically 18 of the 30 publications warned readers that without an abstinence amendment, USAID, which has a "history of anti-abstinence programs," would "garner exorbitant funding" for condom distribution (CWA, March 31, 2003). For good measure, eight publications also made explicit reference to abortion, prostitution and/or homosexuals, establishing a time-tested rhetorical link between their lobbying goals and classic, lurid images of moral decay. "Homosexual groups and pro-abortionist organizations," TVC warned, "are fighting to make certain this legislation becomes simply another condom giveaway program" (TVC, April 25, 2003).

Similarly, 15 of the 30 publications argued that faith-based partners have been discriminated against and that without a conscience-clause they will be shut out of funding opportunities, or forced to distribute condoms against their will. "The problem," wrote Chuck Colson in a BP article, "is that Congress wants faith-based solutions, but without the faith that makes the solution possible [. . .] So we need an amendment that makes it clear faith-based groups can hire people who believe what they believe and not hire people who don't" (BP, April 30, 2003). To make this point more urgently, four of the six special-interest groups argued that the Catholic Church cares for one in four AIDS victims and stood to lose all its money without special protection, an argument completely without merit yet still rhetorically effective. "In fact, one out of every four organizations treating AIDS patients—which are charities—could lose funding because of the lack of conscience protection in the bill" (FoF, April 25, 2003).

Congress and rhetoric on government regulation

Similar to the arguments made by lobbyists, a theme running through Congressional debates was a perception that USAID needed tight regulation, that without the amendments, USAID would continue a "condoms-only" approach, in the process discriminating against FBOs. Indeed the premise itself for including an abstinence earmark and a conscience clause—as opposed to writing a few strongly worded findings into the text of the bill—can only be the perceived unreliability (or unwillingness) of USAID to meet conservative recommendations unless bound by law to do so. "The [abstinence] amendment will ensure," Pitts argued, "that these funds save more lives by moving taxpayer dollars away from failed schemes of the past and to life-saving strategies that have proven to save lives" (IR, April 2, 2003).

Similarly, seven different lawmakers would rise throughout the debates to insist that FBOs have in the past encountered discrimination, and that without revision, the Global AIDS Bill would disqualify religious entities from eligibility for funds. Some of these arguments, identical to those advanced by lobbyists, made unmerited yet persuasive reference to how the Catholic

Church cares for one in four AIDS patients. "The Catholic Church," argued Pitts, "which may have a conscientious objection to distributing condoms, cares for one in four AIDS patients around the world. To deny them funding would be to ignore a crucial partner in the fight against AIDS" (ibid.). In more extreme instances, lawmakers such as Smith (R-NJ) rose to give specific examples of antireligious biases displayed by USAID.

Whether or not the fears articulated here by Republican lawmakers were indeed supported by history or facts is something I was not able to confirm. But they certainly struck a chord with conservatives who had nurtured long-standing suspicions of foreign aid in general and USAID in particular, and it would not be the last time in PEPFAR's lifespan that USAID would come under sustained, heavy criticism from both religious lobbyists and lawmakers.

Conclusions

Vergari (2001, p. 205) argues that some researchers have traditionally specified "two models of the policymaking process: 1) the model of quiet, insider interest-group politics; and 2) the morality politics model exemplified by high salience and broad public participation." The legislative process of ABY, however, appears to have been something of a hybrid between these two models. Although abstinence promotion was lobbied for on the basis of "first principles" and moral values, the defining feature of morality politics, it also involved the extensive and effective participation of Christian interest groups.

The strategy of these interest groups, however, did not fit the traditional model of "outsider tactics" attributed to religious lobbyists in the literature. The case of ABY instead suggests that religious lobbyists employed a sophisticated "insider-outsider" strategy to effect policy change. On the inside they collaborated with allies in Congress to testify at hearings, compose amendments, liaise with lawmakers, and stay abreast of a bill's evolution through Congress's various committees and debates. On the outside they marshaled their membership base through "action alerts" and publicationswhich then pressured Congressmen from the "bottom" with phone calls, e-mails, and faxes. Religious lobbyists also used their access to the executive office and to President Bush, pressuring Congress from the "top."

Although clearly driven by an ideology of Christian sexual morality, a key feature of the interest-group strategy for the Global AIDS Bill was to "demoralize" the abstinence issue by using the functional arguments that abstinence has been "proven to work" in Uganda. The effectiveness of special-interest groups may also be related to the nature of the Global AIDS Bill itself, which did not concern US interests but rather described a foreign policy aimed largely at Africa. In other words, it is possible that interest groups played a uniquely prominent role in this instance of morality policy simply because the general public was neither motivated nor informed enough to participate in an issue concerning Africans.

As a consequence of the hybrid nature of the legislative process, it appears Congress was incentivized to pass a bill that contained significant functional shortcomings. Rather than focus on instrumental concerns about which HIV prevention policies would work, and how both the House and Senate instead passed expressive policies catering to the strongly voiced preferences of religious political actors, thus fulfilling what Cigler and Loomis (2007, p. 30) warn can be the tyranny of the minority:

> [. . .] the American constitutional system is extraordinarily susceptible to the excesses of minority faction—in an ironic way a potential victim of the "Madisonian" solution of dealing with the tyranny of the majority. Decentralized government, especially one that wields considerable power, provides no adequate controls over the excessive demands of interest group politics. Decision makers feel obliged to respond to many of these demands, and "the cumulative effect of this pressure has been the relentless and extraordinary rise of government spending and inflationary deficits, as well as the frustration of efforts to enact effective national policies on most major issues." (Ladd, 1980)

The operative word in the passage above is "effective." Lawmakers altered the Global AIDS Bill without exploring the potential effectiveness of the amendments, leaving questions about implementation, outcomes, and impact to be answered outside Congress.

Questions for reflection

1. How was morality politics used in this case to encourage specific HIV/AIDS legislation?
2. What aspects of this policy were "demoralized" to encourage legislation? How?
3. How do special-interest groups take part in the HIV/AIDS education of politicians?
4. What is the nature of the relationship between democracy (especially free speech) and HIV/AIDS policy? How is HIV/AIDS education policy framed by politics?

Reference list

Blankenau, J., and M. Leeper (2003). "Public school search policies and the 'politics of sin'." *Policy Studies Journal* 31 (4): 565–84.

BP (March 17, 2003). "The African AIDS crisis." Retrieved August 5, 2008, from www.breakpoint.org/listingarticle.asp?ID=5223.

— (April 30, 2003). "Africa's AIDS crisis: the response of a compassionate conservative." Retrieved August 5, 2008, from www.breakpoint.org/listingarticle.asp?id=5510.

— (May 14, 2003). "Bringing down the numbers." Retrieved August 5, 2008, from www.breakpoint.org/listingarticle.asp?ID=5513.

Blumenthal. M. (2009). *Republican Gomorrah: Inside the Movement That Shattered the Party.* New York: Nation Books.

Cigler, A. J., and B. A. Loomis (2007). "Introduction: the changing nature of interest group politics." In A. J. Cigler and B. A. Loomis (eds), *Interest Group Politics.* Washington, DC: CQ Press: 26–8.

Cooperman, A. (2003). "Evangelical Christians lobby for AIDS funds; groups endorse Bush's $15 billion program." *Washington Post*, June 13: A02.

CR (May 1, 2003). "Congressional Record, proceedings and debates of the 108th Congress, 1st session. 149:64." Retrieved August 5, 2008, from http://frwebgate.access.gpo.gov/cgi-bin/getpage.cgi?dbname=2003_record&page=H3573&position=all.

— (May 13, 2003). "Congressional Record, proceedings and debates of the 108th Congress, 1st session. 149:71". Retrieved August 5, 2008, from http://frwebgate2.access.gpo.gov/cgi-bin/PDFgate.cgi?WAISdocID=050806318245+0+1+0&WAISaction=retrieve.

— (May 21, 2003). "Congressional Record, proceedings and debates of the 108th Congress, 1st session. 149:76." Retrieved August 5, 2008, from http://frwebgate.access.gpo.gov/cgi-bin/getpage.cgi?dbname=2003_record&page=H4371&position=all.

Crowley, M. (2004). "James Dobson: the religious right's new kingmaker." Retrieved August 5, 2008, from www.slate.com/id/2109621/.

CWA (March 31, 2003). "AIDS funding: a good idea gone miserably bad?" Retrieved August 5, 2008, from www.beverlylahayeinstitute.org/articledisplay.asp?id=3645&department=BLI&categoryid=femfacts.

— (April 9, 2003). "Beware House Global AIDS Bill." Retrieved 5 August 2008, from www.cwfa.org/printerfriendly.asp?id=3712&department=cfi&categoryid=cfreport.

— (April 30, 2003). "Republicans extol amended AIDS bill." Retrieved 5 August 2008, from www.cultureandfamily.org/articledisplay.asp?id=3879&department=CFI&categoryid=cfrepo.

— (May 1, 2003). "Victory: U.S. House votes to send life, not death, to Africa." Retrieved August 5, 2008, from www.cwfa.org/articledisplay.asp?id=3887&department=MEDIA&categoryid=life.

— (May 15, 2003). "CWA warns delay equals death: Hyde/Lantos Global AIDS Bill must pass immediately with no amendments." Retrieved August 5, 2008, from www.cwfa.org/articledisplay.asp?id=3964&department=MEDIA&categoryid=life.

— (May 16, 2003). "CWA praises swift Senate passage of lifesaving AIDS bill." Retrieved August 5, 2008, from www.cwfa.org/articledisplay.asp?id=3974&department=MEDIA&categoryid=life.

— (May 19, 2003). "African AIDS relief bill passes." Retrieved August 5, 2008, from www.cwfa.org/articles/3976/CWA/family/index.htm.

Eckstrom, K. (2003). "Bush rallies support for aids relief bill." Retrieved August 5, 2008, from pewforum.org/news/display.php?NewsID=2200.

EF (2003a). "Global AIDS Bill letter to President Bush" (April 16). Retrieved August 5, 2008, from www.eagleforum.org/alert/2003/Global-AIDS-bill-Letter.PDF.

— (2003b). "Tell Congress to pass science-based, pro-family amendments to AIDS bill" (April 16). Retrieved August 5, 2008, from www.eagleforum.org/alert/2003/AIDS-4-29-03.shtml.

Figart, N. (2003). "The war on condoms is a war on sex." Retrieved August 5, 2008, from www.mountainpridemedia.org/oitm/issues/2003/07jul2003/views01_figart.htm.

FoF (March 18, 2003). "Troubling Global AIDS Bill looms." Retrieved August 5, 2008, from www.cwfa.org/articles/3575/CFI/cfreport/index.htm.

— (April 15, 2003). "Addressing the African AIDS crisis." Retrieved August 5, 2008, from www.citizenlink.org/CLFeatures/A000000578.cfm.

— (April 25, 2003). "Addressing the African AIDS crisis." Retrieved August 5, 2008, from www.citizenlink.org/CLFeatures/A000000578.cfm.

— (May 16, 2003). "Victory declared on Global AIDS Bill." Retrieved August 5, 2008, from www.citizenlink.org/CLFeatures/A000000574.cfm.

— (October 13, 2003). "Global AIDS Bill in jeopardy." Retrieved August 5, 2008, from www.citizenlink.org/CLFeatures/A000000541.cfm.

— (October 31, 2003). "Feinstein AIDS bill amendment defeated." Retrieved August 5, 2008, from www.citizenlink.org/CLFeatures/A000000536.cfm.

Fowler, R. B., A. D. Hertzke, and L. R. Olson. (1999). *Religion and Politics in America : Faith, Culture, and Strategic Choices*. Boulder, CO: Westview Press.

Gilgoff, D. (2007). *The Jesus Machine : How James Dobson, Focus on the Family, and Evangelical America Are Winning the Culture War*. New York: St. Martin's Press.

Goggin, M., and C. Z. Mooney (2001). "Congressional use of policy information on fact and value issues." In C. Z. Mooney (ed.), *The Public Clash of Private Values: The Politics of Morality Policy*. New York: Chatham House.

Guth, J., L., L. A. Kellstedt, C. E. Smidt, and J. C. Green. (2007). "Getting the spirit? Religious and partisan mobilization in the 2004 elections." In A. J. Cigler, and B. A. Loomis (eds), *Interest Group Politics*. Washington, DC: CQ Press.

Haider-Markel, D. P. (2001). "Morality in congress? Legislative voting on gay issues." In C. Z. Mooney (ed.), *The Public Clash of Private Values: The Politics of Morality Policy*. New York: Chatham House.

Haider-Markel, D. P., and K. Meier (1996). "The politics of gay and lesbian rights: expanding the scope of the conflict." *The Journal of Politics* 58 (2): 332–49.

Hertzke, A. D. (1988). *Representing God in Washington : the Role of Religious Lobbies in the American Polity*. Knoxville: University of Tennessee Press.

Hutcheson, R. G. (1989). *God in the White House: How Religion Has Changed the Modern Presidency*. New York: Collier Books.

IR (2003). "Markup before the Committee on International Relations, House of Representatives, 108th Congress, first session on H.R. 1298" (April 2). Retrieved August 5, 2008, from www.foreignaffairs. house.gov/archives/108/86302.pdf.

Ladd, E. C. (1980). "How to tame the special-interest groups." *Fortune* 102 (8): 66–68.

Mooney, C. Z. (2001). *The Public Clash of Private Values: The Politics of Morality Policy.* New York: Chatham House.

Neuhaus, R. J. and M. Cromartie. [eds] (1987). *Piety and Politics : Evangelicals and Fundamentalists Confront the World.* Washington, DC: Lanham, MD: Ethics and Public Policy Center.

Norrander, B., and C. Wilcox (2001). "Public opinion and policymaking in the States: the case of post-Roe abortion policy." In C. Z. Mooney (ed.), *The Public Clash of Private Values: The Politics of Morality Policy.* New York: Chatham House.

Pierce, P., and D. Miller (2001). "Variations in the diffusion of state lottery adoptions: how revenue dedication changes morality politics." In C. Z. Mooney (ed.), *The Public Clash of Private Values: The Politics of Morality Policy.* New York: Chatham House.

Schuman, J. (1998). "Religious right makes stand against GOP." Associated Press press release (May 9). Retrieved June 20, 2008, from www.positiveatheism.org/writ/flaplate.htm#DOBSONVGOP.

Sharlet, J. (2006). "God's senator: who would Jesus vote for? Meet Sam Brownback." Retrieved June 21, 2008, from www.rollingstone.com/politics/story/9178374/gods_senator.

TVC (April 25, 2003). "AIDS legislation still needs amendments." Retrieved August 5, 2008, from www. traditionalvalues.org/modules.php?sid=889.

— (October 16, 2003). "Global AIDS Bill in jeopardy." Retrieved August 5, 2008, from www. traditionalvalues.org/modules.php?sid=1242.

— (October 31, 2003). "Global AIDS Bill saved from Feinstein amendment." Retrieved August 5, 2008, from www.traditionalvalues.org/modules.php?sid=1279.

USGov (2003). "'United States Leadership Act Against HIV/AIDS, Tuberculosis, and Malaria Act of 2003. Public law no. 108–25, 117 Stat. 711." Retrieved April 14, 2008, from http://frwebgate.access. gpo.gov/cgi-bin/getdoc.cgi?dbname=108_cong_bills&docid=f:h1298enr.txt.pdf.

Vergari, S. (2001). "Morality politics and the implementation of abstinence-only sex education: a case of policy compromise." In C. Z. Mooney (ed.), *The Public Clash of Private Values: The Politics of Morality Policy.* New York: Chatham House.

Health Promotion through ABC Education: Agenda Setting and the Development of the ABC Strategy in Zambia

3

Doreen Tembo

Chapter Outline

Introduction

The way national policy regarding an HIV/AIDS prevention strategy is created and implemented can have a significant impact on its success or failure. One of the most influential and debated HIV prevention strategies employed around the world has been health education based on the Abstinence–Be faithful–Condom Use (ABC) approach. However, there are different substrategies that exist within the ABC strategy, which have each shown levels of success. For instance, *abstinence* can refer to primary abstinence, or delaying, or never engaging in sex. It can also refer to secondary abstinence (deciding to abstain after previously engaging in sex) and *being faithful* can imply monogamy, reducing casual sex, reducing the number of sexual partners, or fidelity within polygamous unions, and *condom use* should ideally imply correct and consistent use of male or female condoms.

Ugandan national policy, which is often credited as successful because of its use of the ABC strategy, focused on abstinence or delaying sex before marriage and mutual fidelity, while condoms were advocated for those who were unwilling to abstain or be faithful. The "success" of this strategy (HIV prevalence fell from around 15 percent in the early 1990s to about 5 percent in 2001), however, may have had help from other factors in the Ugandan context. In order to explore the causes for this reduction in prevalence, researchers have identified contextual factors including:

- rates of monogamy
- partner reduction
- delayed sexual debut
- condom use
- social mobilization
- positive involvement of people living with HIV/AIDS (PLWHA)
- religious leaders and faith-based organizations (FBOs) in the HIV/AIDS response
- care and support for PLWHA
- increased positive interpersonal discourse at the community level
- raised social status of women
- high-level political support
- a multisectoral response
- a decentralized planning and implementation program
- policy addressing HIV-related stigma and discrimination
- voluntary counseling and testing (VCT)
- condom promotion

While it may be impossible to pinpoint just why prevalence declined in the case of Uganda, we can explore other contexts in which the ABC strategy was used and less success was reported and try to understand what factors contributed to this "failure."

Zambia had been included among other countries, which were claimed to have, like Uganda, successfully lowered new HIV infection rates because of the use of the ABC strategy. HIV prevalence, casual sex, and multiple sexual partnerships during the late 1990s had fallen in Zambia (Agha, 2002; Bessinger et al., 2003; Fylkesnes et al., 2001), but only by 1.3 percent between 2001 and 2007. Currently at 15.2 percent, Zambia still has one of the highest rates of new HIV infections in the world (UNAIDS, 2008).

Though Zambia and Uganda are relatively close in geography, share similar cultural, economic, and political contexts compared to the rest of the world, and seem to have a similar timeline of HIV/AIDS policy action, the results are much different. How can we learn from the Zambian experience about what impacts the success of an educational strategy?

This chapter presents findings from a case study of the Zambian government's agenda-setting process for the ABC strategy within the wider agenda-setting process for the HIV/AIDS prevention policy. Using a public-policy analysis framework developed by Knoepfel et al. (2007), this chapter narrates the timeline of AIDS policy with a focus on the rise of the ABC strategy between 1986, at the start of the HIV/AIDS epidemic, and 2005 when the National HIV/AIDS policy was formalized in the Zambian parliament. This framework analyzes the interaction between actors, the resources available to policy actors, and the general institutional rules governing all policies as well as the institutional rules specific to the policy under study at each stage of the policy cycle. It also examines the policy outputs at each stage, while taking into account the prevailing economic, political, and social developments in the country.

The narrative presented in this chapter comes from a literature review, qualitative content analysis (QCA) of health-sector and HIV/AIDS policy documents, and interviews with policy makers and implementers between 2005 and 2006. These key informants were often leaders of organizations or agencies dealing with HIV/AIDS policy, or were the primary HIV/AIDS policy leaders within organizations or agencies. The content of these interviews as well as of the literature review and the QCA were analyzed using the qualitative analysis software program NVIVO. The themes derived from this analysis are presented in this chapter utilizing a historical analysis in conjunction with Knoepfel et al.'s (2007) policy analysis framework. Results from this analysis show how the various actors, the resources available to them, the culture of the society at large and the specific institutions in which these actors worked all impacted the ABC strategy's formation and implementation and could have led to the strategy's relatively unsuccessful results.

Did an early biomedical response miss chances to implement a comprehensive ABC strategy?

In 1986, increasing AIDS-related deaths and bed occupancy in hospitals led the Ministry of Health (MoH) and the World Health Organization (WHO Program on AIDS) to identify HIV and AIDS as a medical rather than a social or political problem. The problem was thus not immediately taken up in the policy agenda and the focus of the 1986 First Emergency Short-Term Plan was solely on the prevention of blood-supply and blood-product contamination (Republic of Zambia, 2005, p. 8). The 1988–92 First Medium-Term Plan continued to treat the epidemic as a biomedical problem, and HIV/AIDS prevention efforts were consolidated with other opportunist infections (OI) such as tuberculosis (TB) and leprosy as well as with STIs, which facilitate HIV transmission. The 1988–92 First Medium-Term Plan prioritized a total of eight areas: TB and leprosy; information, education, and communication (IEC); counseling; laboratory support; epidemiology and research; STIs and clinical care; program management and home-based care (Republic of Zambia, 2005 [University of Zambia interview], p. 8). Although IEC was a priority, interviews with the Ministry of Education revealed that a clear comprehensive prevention message was not disseminated to the public.

The prevailing social, economic, and political environment influenced the lack of a comprehensive ABC prevention message in the official IEC strategy at this early stage of the epidemic. During this early response to the epidemic, the Zambian economy was still in a state of decline due to the 1970s oil crisis and the fall in copper prices. The state was in conflict with international aid agencies (notably the International Monetary Fund and World Bank), which had imposed economic structural adjustment programs in exchange for access to their funds (Saasa and Carlsson, 1996). Because of the country's colonial history, the state (United National Independence Party) was especially resentful of efforts by external international agencies to provide monetary and technical aid for family planning (including condom promotion). Politicians viewed the promotion of family planning by international organizations such as the United Nations Population Fund (UNFPA), the United Nations Children's Fund (UNICEF) and the World Health Organization (WHO) as part of the "white man's efforts to control the growth of the black population" rather than as legitimate development efforts (Solo et al., 2005, p. vii; Walt, et al., 1999a). Public discussion of sexual issues is considered taboo in Zambian society and, given the agrarian nature of economic activity, the low socioeconomic status of women, and the state-wide predominance of far-right Christian ideology, it was not surprising that a pronatalist ideology was favored and family planning was very unpopular, even controversial (Nanda, 2000). As such, political commitment to family planning programs was low and many of the reproductive health programs including family planning and STI control programs were run by nongovernmental organizations (NGOs) such as the Family Planning Welfare Association of Zambia and the Planned Parenthood Association of Zambia (PPAZ).

It is unsurprising that the MoH, through the National HIV/AIDS Prevention and Control Program, did not include messages about condom use (a contraceptive as well as prophylaxis) or clearly provide comprehensive information about HIV/AIDS in its early public-health promotion campaigns in hospitals and schools. The public where thus not given a clear, informed strategy for avoiding infection; instead HIV/AIDS was viewed as something to be feared and abstinence was advocated as the only safe option. According to interviews conducted at the Ministry of Education and the University of Zambia, many of these messages were authoritarian and promoted through fear by representing HIV/AIDS through cartoons of emaciated AIDS patients, predatory birds, or dark shadowy figures with messages such as "sex, thrills, AIDS kills."

This represented a missed opportunity for a clear message that would have decreased stigma through encouraging positive and informed discussion of HIV/AIDS in communities and social networks, as well as promoting condom use as a state-backed prevention method. Advocating abstinence for young and unmarried people, and especially girls, and fidelity for women was a cultural and religious norm in Zambia (Rasing, 2003; Taylor, 2006). In the tradition of targeting reproductive health activities mainly at children and women (Lush et al., 1999), HIV-prevention messages were mostly in schools and antenatal clinics and hospitals. These early messages failed to reach and engage men, the real power brokers in Zambian homes. Because extramarital relationships are reported to be especially prevalent among men in Zambia (Halperin and Epstein, 2004; Central Statistical Office et al., 2009), not reaching men with partner reduction or fidelity messages, at this early stage, represented a missed opportunity for HIV prevention.

The start of the HIV/AIDS epidemic was thus characterized by the promotion of the "A" and "B" messages by local actors (the state and FBOs) as well as societal institutional rules, especially targeting women and children. Meanwhile the "C" message was supported mostly by foreign international actors and local NGOs. Relations between the state and international actors took a turn for the worse when the state refused to conform to SAP conditions leading to the freezing of funds by all major international aid agencies just a month before the election in 1991 (Blas and Limbambala, 2001a; Lake and Musumali, 1999. This deterioration in relations opened a door for a select few international aid organizations to expand funding directly or vertically to local NGOs. Through the newly established Society for Family Health (SFH) and the pre-existing PPAZ, international aid agencies, such as USAID, increased their direct support to reproductive health services. Social marketing of condoms by the SFH began as early as 1992, and the SFH came to be responsible for more than one third of all condoms available in the market (Solo et al., 2005). A further shift in actor dynamics and institutional culture and rules was to come when the Movement for Multiparty Democracy (MMD) party won the election in 1991.

The path-dependent nature of societal institutional rules

The MMD party, driven by an ideological neoliberal economic ethos, aimed to restructure the state and fully implement the SAP with a special focus on the single largest cause of government expenditure: the health sector and reproductive health services (Blas and Limbambala, 2001b; Cassel and Janowski, 1996; Jeppsson and Okuonzi, 2000; MoH, 1992; Nanda, 1999; Walt et al., 1999b). The early government enjoyed affable relations with international organizations as their ethos mirrored that of key development-centered international agencies. The healthcare reforms as outlined in the 1994 National Strategic Plan centered on improving leadership, accountability within the health sector, and partnership with the different health sector actors (Lake and Musumali, 1999; MoH, 1992). Partnerships, collaboration, and coordination between the state, international aid agencies, international NGOs, and civil society (defined here as local NGOs, community-based organizations [CBOs] and faith-based organizations [FBOs]) were encouraged. The government introduced the sector-wide approach (SWAp) to management of health programs and coordination of resources in 1993. The SWAp aimed to increase the ability of government to manage healthcare by discouraging the vertical funding of projects and organizations and instead encouraging aid agencies to contribute to one central fund. (Bennett, 1998). The state and aid agencies would thereafter consultatively devise strategic plans and activities which would have to be approved by government, only thereafter would funds to smaller projects or organizations be allocated.

Reproductive health reform, including the improvement of the status of women and reproductive and sexual health services (contraception), was given greater impetus by the Zambian state's commitment to the resolutions and program of action of the 1994 International Conference on Population and Development (ICPD) and the 1995 Beijin Platform for Action (Mayhew et al., 2000).

Changes to the policy-making process were instituted by the new MMD government. In 1993, the Policy Analysis and Coordination Division were established in the Cabinet Office to design and implement the policy-formulation and implementation process. The policy-making process shifted from a centrally administered, heavily bureaucratic, rule-driven one, to a more democratic, coordinated, consultative, decentralized, and monitored process.

As predicted by dynamic models of policy analysis, it was expected that these sudden and unexpected changes in the general and specific institutional rules, the relationship between the state and international aid organizations, partnerships with civil society, reproductive health policy and service provision, and the policy-making process would lead to HIV/AIDS being taken on to the political policy agenda (Baumgartner and Jones, 1993). The strategy toward HIV/AIDS had thus far been developed using a top-down approach and HIV/AIDS was still being treated as a biomedical problem by the "owning" ministry, the MoH. However HIV/AIDS had not been defined as a problem by communities where, according to the interview with the University of Zambia, "people still feared HIV/AIDS and did not speak about it." The first HIV/AIDS prevention program by the MMD government, the Second Mid-term Plan (1994–98) was launched in 1993, and it integrated prevention and care efforts for AIDS, TB and STIs (as well as leprosy). This was the first plan to specifically mention the need to promote condoms, yet the Second Mid-term Plan did not explicitly explore the related strategies. NGOs such as the SFH and the PPAZ remained in the forefront of condom promotion to the public while the MoH promoted these in health institutions.

The low levels of political commitment to HIV/AIDS prevention that characterized the period covered by the Second Mid-term Plan largely accounted for the lack of state-backed promotion of condoms (National HIV/AIDS/STI/TB Council, 2000), and interviews and literature strongly indicate that political attitudes toward condom promotion were especially hostile during this same period. Although state-related institutional rules had shifted in favor of condom promotion, the societal institutional rules remained unchanged. Culturally sensitive or right-wing, Christian politicians (including the president) and religious organizations were reluctant to promote the use of condoms despite research-proven success (Garbus, 2003; Pinkerton and Abramson, 1997; Weller, 1993). An official with the Ministry of Education reflected, "Sometimes it all depends on the political relationship we have at any given time. We had a minister that was a reverend and did not want to appear to support anything to do with condoms" (MoE interview,2006).

Interviews at the University of Zambia (UNZA) highlighted how some of the Christian far-right members of government campaigned to ban condom commercials, questioned their efficacy, and stopped distribution in public institutions (especially in schools and prisons). The 1990s came to be characterized by constant conflict between far-right Christian groups and politicians on one hand and health-care professionals, NGOs, and the donor groups promoting condoms on the other (Mouli, 1992).

By the end of the Second Mid-term Plan (1994–98), a review of the government's response by multiorganizational stakeholders (including government, WHO, and UNAIDS), conducted between June 1998 and June 1999, found the government's response unsatisfactory. A second report funded by the independent UK Department for International Development (DFID) came to similar conclusions.

The influence of international actors and resources in the policy process

The National HIV/AIDS/ST/TB Council (NAC) was established by parliament in 2000 to address the concerns documented in these two reports. NAC was to coordinate government and civil society, provide leadership and policy guidance, and mobilize resources for the HIV/AIDS response. The creation of

NAC was largely a UNAIDS-led initiative; NAC's structure and operational remit was very similar to the Ugandan AIDS commission (established in 1992) and to UNAIDS itself (established in 1996), as reflected in the "three ones" approach (one national AIDS framework, one national AIDS authority, and one system for monitoring and evaluation) that was developed and used by UNAIDS. Further, major funding for HIV prevention and care programs, such as the World Bank's Country AIDS Program, was only disbursed on condition that countries requesting aid had an overall coordinating body ("housed in the highest level of state government") as well as a national strategic plan and a commitment to disburse between 40 to 60 percent of funds to civil society (Görgens-Albino, *et al.*, 2007). Several interviewed policy makers and implementers pointed out that while Zambia was very good at policy borrowing, in this case largely from UNAIDS and Uganda, it was either not committed to these borrowed policies or did not have enough resources to implement them.

International agencies indirectly affected all key elements of the policy analytic framework as well as policy outputs. That is, the availability of vital resources were only going to be made available to the state when the state complied with changes in its institutional rules (the creation of NAC), its network of policy actors (through a more thorough inclusion of civil society), and the creation of a national policy. The conditions imposed by international aid agencies brought HIV/AIDS onto the political agenda as NAC was to be "housed in the highest level of state government", or in the case of Zambia, the cabinet committee of ministers who directly reported to the head of state. Despite this documentary evidence of the coercive power of international aid agencies, interviewees at international agencies and state ministries strongly insisted that policy direction and inspiration came from the state and that international agencies only provided technical support. However, when asked about where policy *direction* came from, an interview with a MoH official revealed that policy could be "donor driven."

It took two years for NAC to be established as a legal body with the ability to solicit and raise its own funds by an act of parliament through the 2002 National AIDS Bill. This perhaps reflects the fact that NAC was not a wholly government-led initiative but was created to satisfy donor conditions and technical advice from UNAIDS. Furthermore, the majority of the interviewed policy makers and implementers pointed out that NAC was a good idea in principle but was too understaffed and underfunded to effectively coordinate the response. Despite the introduction of SWAp, encouraging international aid to be funneled through a single channel, one interview with a representative of NAC highlighted how civil society organizations were still not using NAC as their primary source of funding, and were still predominantly vertically funded by outside agencies. This made it difficult for NAC to control their direction or to evaluate their outcomes. It also created competition between the state and NGOs (Geloo, 2004), and decreased collaboration and coordination of HIV/AIDS prevention strategies causing a duplication of programs and an inefficient use of scarce resources. Although NAC is supposed to improve this situation, it has also been criticized for being more interested in acquiring resources rather than implementing measures to strengthen coordination. In an interview with a SHARE official, the following statement was made:

> The council was established and now there's still a lot of disagreement. People want to start writing cheques; they want to control funding, and decide who gets what money. It's a distraction. That shouldn't be the primary function of the National AIDS Council. It's spending time and finding out who needs what support, and effective coordination. That is what the National AIDS Council is supposed to be doing. It has achieved some success but there is a lot more to be done.

An expanded network of policy actors moves toward a comprehensive ABC strategy

Despite these reported problems between policy actors, HIV/AIDS was finally on the political agenda. The framework developed for 2001–3 reflected the state's efforts to restructure the HIV/AIDS policy and programming as a response to the critiques in the two reports by UNAIDS/WHO and DFID. Because of this re-evaluation, there was a delay in NAC becoming operational. Meanwhile the MoH, through its Zambian National AIDS/STD/TB and Leprosy Program (NASTLP), remained responsible for the policy formulation and production of the 2001–3 national framework. The MoH would later provide guidance for the formulation and operationalization of NAC.

Although the MoH was the main lead organization in the development of the 2001–3 HIV/AIDS strategic framework, there was a change in the larger set of actors working on this policy. Between 1998 and 1999, the working group consisted of 2 members from the NASTLP, while the rest of the 12 members and 3 resource staff came from UN organizations, NGOs, FBOs, key health projects, the Network of Zambian People Living with HIV/AIDS and the Ministry of Finance and Economic Development (now the Ministry of Finance and National Planning). One UNZA official reported:

> This (HIV/AIDS) was seen as an issue of the MoH. Now when we look at HIV/AIDS in the framework of a multisectoral response, it wasn't only the ministry's responsibility to respond to HIV/AIDS, it was everybody's responsibility.

The interview at UNZA revealed that the initial biomedical response to HIV/AIDS meant that HIV/AIDS was "lumped" with a host of different diseases including STDs, tuberculosis (TB) and leprosy. When compared to TB, which is one of the most common opportunistic infections linked to AIDS, and STIs which facilitate transmission of HIV, leprosy itself has a weak association with the epidemic (Corbett et al., 2003; Pilcher et al., 2004; Ustianowski et al., 2006). The 2001–3 strategic framework removed leprosy from the remit of the HIV/AIDS response, signaling a more streamlined HIV/AIDS response.

The content of the 2001–3 strategic framework also fitted into the country's overall economic development program and aimed to encourage foreign bilateral and multilateral debt cancellation to better mitigate the effects of the pandemic, reflecting the political agenda of this government (Mwikisa, 2002; National HIV/AIDS/STI/TB Council, 2000). The budgetary costs of implementing the 2001–3 framework demonstrated that there would be a deficit of 68 percent after accounting for both government and aid agencies' funding. The budget thus demonstrated that it would be impossible for the government to fully implement the framework under the prevailing levels of external debt repayment and foreign aid.

> The framework is also written in the context of a possible "debt for development swap." The Government of Zambia has been carrying out careful planning of how monies saved from interest payments on foreign loans could serve the purposes of poverty reduction, education, reducing the impact of AIDS and other social goals. (NAC, 2000, p. iii)

The ABC strategy was more fully promoted as a priority intervention in the 2001–3 framework after the policy network was dominated by actors from local and international civil society, representatives from PLWHA networks, and technical advisors from the UN. The 2001–3 framework identified elements of the ABC strategy as a primary goal, defined in the framework as "behavior change: abstinence, mutual faithfulness, or condom use," and "reduction of high-risk behavior" (e.g. multiple partners). However this framework did not explicitly specify *how* the ABC strategy was going to be implemented and evaluated. Instead, it was to be *implicitly* advocated through a variety of targeted interventions. The promotion of condoms was only explicitly listed as a "strategic goal of best practice" for "high-risk" groups and not the general population. Nor were abstinence and mutual fidelity explicitly mentioned.

One of the policy goals in this framework was to identify and expand successful evidence-based or "catalytic" projects. Many of these projects were being run by NGOs funded by foreign bodies. Only about 40 percent of these projects were being implemented by a government institution or agency alone or in coordination with another organization. The new plan assigned a government ministry to each one of the catalytic projects. In a similar vein, the 2002 Zambia Poverty Reduction Paper (PRP) prominently featured the reduction of HIV/AIDS through a multisectoral approach that promoted behavior change through IEC as a first level priority. The PRP also advocated the expansion of effective programs already being run by civil society. The PRP document urged increased collaboration with NGOs, CBOs, and communities to effect behavior change. HIV/AIDS policy was clearly brought to the political agenda through the participation of civil society and international organizations in the policy process as well as the government's desire for debt relief. These factors also increased political action by challenging the religious and cultural institutional rules that were impeding the successful implementation of full ABC promotion (as opposed to partial), propelling policy towards more evidence-based interventions.

Tackling ABC-related societal institution rules and legislature

Even as the state was turning its attention toward changing the institutional rules and policy guiding HIV/AIDS prevention, there was also an effort to change the negative societal rules that impeded the successful implementation of the ABC strategy. National campaigns that sought to challenge harmful social institutional rules, such as the taboo of speaking openly about sex and promoting contraception (including condoms), were implemented. Civil society and international agencies had been running projects that encouraged community and traditional leaders to participate in promoting HIV prevention and risk-reducing behaviors in the 1990s. For example, traditional leaders in the southern province of Zambia substituted sexual rites that increased risk of HIV transmission with nonsexual rites (Malungo, 2001).

A major USAID-supported ABC campaign (called HEART), designed for youth in partnership with youth, was broadcast beginning in 2001. It promoted delayed sexual debut and increased abstinence while still educating youth about condoms (Olson and Population Services International, 2003; Underwood et al., 2006). A major campaign promoting acceptance of people living with HIV/AIDS, VCT, and ABC utilized prominent political figures (including the first president of Zambia, Dr. Kenneth Kaunda), traditional chiefs and popular musicians, and was aired between 2002 and 2003 (US Agency for International Development, 2003). Media sources indicate that while religious leaders strongly opposed these campaigns, a new public discourse about HIV/AIDS helped to fight against the "culture of silence" regarding these taboo topics (IRIN PlusNews and UN Office for the Coordination of Humanitarian Affairs, 2002).

One of the key criticisms of the prevention efforts made prior to 2000 was the lack of gender mainstreaming in prevention programs. The success of behavior-change programs that targeted women, especially commercial sex workers, was being impeded by not addressing traditional gender roles where men often took greater power (Campbell and Kelly, 1995; Mbizvo and Bassett, 1996). In launching the Family Planning in Reproductive Health Policy, Framework, Strategies and Guidelines in 1996, the state also followed through with previous commitments to the promotion of gender equality. The development of this policy framework was a consultative process between the state (MoH), civil society, international aid and technical assistance organizations, private sector, and traditional leaders (Bosman et al., 2007). The state then adopted a national policy on gender in 2002 and mainstreamed gender into the Fifth National Development Plan by outlining measures to increase education and economic autonomy among women, and decrease gender-based violence (National HIV/AIDS/STI/TB Council, 2000; Republic of Zambia and Ministry of Foreign Affairs, 2008).

Since 2000, legislative changes to institutional rules have helped to create an environment that supports the implementation of the ABC strategy by passing laws relating to HIV/AIDS discrimination, gender relations, and child protection. The national HIV/AIDS policy has proposed an amendment to the Employment Act, Caption 512, so as to make nonvoluntary HIV pre-screening illegal (Republic of Zambia, 2005). However, this amendment is yet to be made. Section 39 of the draft constitution prohibits discrimination on the basis of "health."

Section 40 of the draft constitution legislates in favor of equal treatment for men and women and Section 44 legislates on equality before, during, and on dissolution of marriage. The Penal Code (Amendment) Act No. 15 of 2005 legislates against marital rape, extends the definition of sexual harassment to include use of sexual imposition through force, legislates against child neglect that endangers the health of the child, and criminalizes cultural practices (including sexual cleansing and female genital mutilation) that may harm a child or perpetuate the transfer of disease. Section 40 of the draft criminalizes laws that undermine the dignity and welfare of women. These changes created a facilitating and favorable environment for the development of the national HIV/AIDS policy.

A comprehensive ABC approach

The 2001–3 strategic framework laid a foundation for a more structured, collaborative, and multisectoral framework to promote evidence-based policies and programs after the National HIV/AIDS/STI/TB Intervention Strategic Plan was produced in 2002. A network of policy actors similar to that of the previous framework worked on this plan, including NAC, civil society, MoH and other government ministries, and international aid and technical assistance organizations. While the 2001–3 framework focused on *planning* the role of the newly formed NAC and the *future direction* of the HIV/AIDS response, the new Intervention Strategic Plan concentrated on implementing both of them.

The Intervention Strategic Plan was innovative in several ways. While it first recognized the comprehensive ABC strategy by endorsing *abstinence* (for youth and unmarried persons), and *fidelity* to one sexual partner, and by discouraging multiple sex partners, it also promoted the universal distribution of affordable *condoms* for general use and not solely in connection with high-risk groups. For the first time, the state called for the public sector to be involved in the wide distribution of condoms. This plan was also the first to offer explicit suggestions on how to reduce concurrent sexual relationships. These suggestions included utilizing marriage counselors and traditional initiators (those who performed sexual initiation and marriage rites) to design culturally sensitive sex education. While empowering women in sexual negotiations was mentioned as a measure to reduce harmful sexual practices, no mention was made of how men were to be engaged.

The Intervention Strategic Plan was also the first to raise the importance of finalizing the national policy and establishing a legal framework for the HIV/AIDS response. Previously, the lack of a national policy had resulted in a redundancy in programs and projects, the underutilization of HIV/AIDS actors, and the waste of scarce health resources. This policy was expected to provide the requisite framework for informing and guiding various stake-holders. Interviews at the MoH revealed that the process of creating a national HIV/AIDS policy had begun as early as 1997. Those involved in the creation of policy mentioned that intensively consulting a large number of actors during the policy-formulation process had caused delays. Differing viewpoints and interests had also created conflict between policy actors, extending the delays further. One MoH official stated:

> We experience a lot of delays, especially on the part of ministers signing off on the document, especially when we have a change in office. Different ministers come with their own political motivations and agendas, and thus they may disagree with what their predecessors might have wanted to be incorporated into the policy; for example, the removal of all homosexual reference. The policy also has to be written in a nontechnical way that can be easily understood; this sometimes can make things complicated as we have to come up with definitions that everyone has to agree on.

The foreword to this policy document reflected the state's desire to comply with the "three ones" approach in order to receive funding from international aid agencies.

The HIV/AIDS policy was finally approved in 2005 and is very similar in its objectives to the 2002–5 plan. The policy is nontechnical and highlights the government's aims, objectives, and measures to achieve these objectives. This time, HIV/AIDS prevention objective did not explicitly advocate abstinence as the best or only method of prevention. Instead, sex education and life-skills training were emphasized for youth. Mutual fidelity was also not explicitly mentioned, although partner reduction is suggested among the measures to reduce STIs. The policy does, however, clearly highlight the objective of making condoms accessible and affordable to all sexually active individuals in the county. Abstinence for the general population of youth and unmarried people is only mentioned in conjunction with the objective to exploit the potential of FBOs in the policy response.

Thus, the final policy represented a shift in ideology from linking specific strategies to certain "risk groups" or gender to encouraging all Zambians to make fully informed choices. Policy had shifted from merely pointing to a limited version of the ABC strategy to promoting and coordinating the use of the full version. This was to change when, in the 2000s, United States of America-based, right-wing political ideology on sexuality tied the US President's Emergency Plan for AIDS Relief (PEPFAR) funding to the condition that recipient countries, which include Zambia and Uganda, spend the majority of the funds on abstinence until marriage (A and B) programs. Smith (2008) reports that Zambia's reliance on PEPFAR funding meant that the new, comprehensive ABC strategy developed at the start of the 2000 decade was being reduced to the A, B and a "silent C" of years past. Although the SWAp system has improved coordination of resources and lessened the coercive power of aid and donor agencies, the system still does not function optimally as donors continue to vertically fund projects and civil society. Thus, despite the development of a detailed ABC strategy and HIV policy framework, the ABC strategy continues to face challenges.

Conclusions

Several macro factors such as economic crisis and debt have substantially determined the severity and scope of the HIV/AIDS epidemic in Zambia. However, within this context, many other variables have impacted the way that the ABC strategy has been incorporated and implemented into national policy. This chapter has attempted to explore these variables, using interviews with many of those officials and representatives of organizations and ministries responsible for this policy, a pervasive literature review, and a qualitative content analysis of documents. The results show that a combination of shifting actors, resources, general and specific formal institutional rules, and societal rules including far-right Christian and traditional views on gender, sex, and contraception all have impacted the ABC strategy in Zambia.

As discussed at the outset, the Ugandan response has been credited as being successful because of the use of the ABC strategy, while many argue that credit is due to a combination of the ABC strategy with the fact that the state and other actors acted swiftly at the start of the epidemic to influence key societal rules such as the social status of women, positively engage with religious groups and men, create open discourse about HIV/AIDS, and decrease stigma. In contrast, while the ABC strategy was technically included in the Zambian HIV/AIDS response from the start, for the majority of the 1990s, the policy arena was characterized by conflict between evidence-based prevention and the traditional or Christian/right-wing moral agendas, especially regarding condoms. Because condom use was, as a result, largely promoted by organizations with international funding, there was a perception, initially, that they were stigmatized as "foreign" intervention. Other complementary efforts to the ABC strategy in Zambia, such as gender mainstreaming and addressing stigma, were also delayed.

Questions for reflection

1. What social, political, and cultural groups impacted the nature of HIV/AIDS education policy in Zambia?
2. How can perceptions about localized versus foreign policies impact HIV/AIDS education?

Reference list

Agha, S. (2002). "An evaluation of the effectiveness of a peer sexual health intervention among secondary-school students in Zambia." *AIDS Education and Prevention* 14(4): 269–81.

Baumgartner, F. and B. Jones, (1993). *Agendas and Instability in American Politics.* Chicago, IL: University of Chicago Press.

Bennett, S. (1999). "Health sector reforms in Zambia: putting them in perspective." In J. Jacobson and J. Bruce (eds), *Report of the Meeting on the Implications of Health Sector Reform on Reproductive Health and Rights: December 14–15, 1998: Washington, D.C.* Takoma Park, MD: Center for Health and Gender Equity, Population Council, pp. 24–8.

Bessinger, R., P. Akwara, and D. Halperin (2003). *Sexual Behaviour, HIV and Fertility Trends: A Comparative Analysis of Six Countries: Phase I of the ABC Study.* Washington, DC: US Agency for International Development.

Blas, E., and M. E. Limbambala (2001a). "The challenge of hospitals in health sector reform: the case of Zambia." *Health Policy and Planning* 16 (SUPPL. 2): 29–43.

— (2001b). "User-payment, decentralization and health service utilization in Zambia." *Health Policy and Planning* 16 (SUPPL. 2): 19–28.

Bosman, M., E. Jongekrijg, and A. Verburg (2007). *A Survey on HIV/AIDS in Zambia.* Retrieved June 2010, from Read:www.prismaweb.org/algemeen/topics/algemeen/documentatie/zambia_hiv_aids_dec_2007.pdf

Campbell, T., and M. Kelly (1995). "Women and AIDS in Zambia: a review of the psychosocial factors implicated in the transmission of HIV." *AIDS Care—Psychological and Socio-Medical Aspects of AIDS/HIV* 7 (3): 365–73.

Cassel, A., and K. Janowski (1996). *Reform of the Health Sector in Ghana and Zambia: Commonalities and Contrasts.* Geneva: World Health Organization.

Central Statistical Office (CSO), Ministry of Health (MOH), Tropical Diseases Research Centre (TDRC), University of Zambia, and Macro International Inc. (2009). *Zambia Demographic and Health Survey, 2007.* Calverton, Maryland: CSO and Macro International.

Corbett, E. L. E. L., Watt, C. J., Walker, N., Maher, D., Williams, B. G., Raviglione, M. C. (2003). "The growing burden of tuberculosis: global trends and interactions with the HIV epidemic." *Archives of Internal Medicine* 163 (9): 1009–21.

Fylkesnes, K. Musonda, R. M., Sichone, M., Ndhlovu, Z., Tembo, F., & Monze, M. (2001). "Declining HIV prevalence and risk behaviours in Zambia: evidence from surveillance and population-based surveys." *AIDS* 15 (7): 907–16.

Garbus, L. (2003). *HIV/AIDS in Zambia*. San Francisco: Country AIDS Policy Analysis Project, AIDS Policy Research Center, University of California San Francisco.

Geloo, Z. (2004). "Health Zambia: NGOs in the hot seat." [Electronic Version]. Inter Press Service News Agency. Retrieved October 24, 2010, from http://ipsnews.net/africa/interna.asp?idnews=22739.

Görgens-Albino, M., N. Mohammad, D.Blankhart, and O. Odutolu (2007). *The Africa Multi-Country AIDS Program 2000–2006*. Washington DC: The International Bank for Reconstruction and Development/The World Bank.

Halperin, D. T., and H. Epstein (2004). "Concurrent sexual partnerships help to explain Africa's high HIV prevalence: implications for prevention." *Lancet* 364 (9428): 4–6.

IRIN PlusNews/UN Office for the Coordination of Humanitarian Affairs (2002). "Zambia: Kaunda soldiers on anti-AIDS campaign." [Electronic Version]. Retrieved October 27, 2010.

Jeppsson, A., and S. A. Okuonzi (2000). "Vertical or holistic decentralization of the health sector? Experiences from Zambia and Uganda." *International Journal of Health Planning and Management* 15 (4): 273–89.

Knoepfel, P., C. Larrue, F. Varone, and M. Hill (2007). *Public Policy Analysis*. Bristol: Policy Press.

Lake, S., and C. Musumali (1999). "Zambia: the role of aid management in sustaining visionary reform." *Health Policy and Planning* 14 (3): 254–63.

Lush, L., J. Cleland, G. Walt, and S. Mayhew (1999). "Integrating reproductive health: myth and ideology." *Bulletin of the World Health Organization* 77 (9): 771–7.

Malungo, J. R. S. (2001). "Sexual cleansing (Kusalazya) and levirate marriage (Kunjilila mung'anda) in the era of AIDS: changes in perceptions and practices in Zambia." *Social Science & Medicine* 53 (3): 371–82.

Mayhew, S. H., L. Lush, J. Cleland, and G. Walt (2000). "Implementing the integration of component services for reproductive health." *Studies in Family Planning* 31 (2): 151–62.

Mbizvo, M. T., and M. T. Bassett (1996). "Reproductive health and AIDS prevention in sub-Saharan Africa: the case for increased male participation." *Health Policy and Planning* 11 (1): 84–92.

Ministry of Health (1992). *National Health Policies and Strategies: Health Reforms*. Lusaka: Government of the Republic of Zambia.

Mouli, V. C. (1992). "Bridges crossed yesterday, peaks to be conquered tomorrow: AIDS and the condom." *Africa Health* 14 (5): 12–14.

Mwikisa, C. N. (2002). "HIV/AIDS interventions in Zambia: financial implications." Paper presented at the 10th General Assembly of CODESRIA.

Nanda, P. (1999). "Global agendas: health sector reforms and reproductive health rights in Zambia." *Development* 42 (4): 59–63.

— (2000). *Health Sector Reforms in Zambia: Implications for Reproductive Health and Rights*. Takoma Park, MD: Centre for Health and Gender Equity

National HIV/AIDS/STI/TB Council (2002). "Official website." Retrieved October 29, 2009, from www.nac.org.zm/index.php/about-us/institutional-framework

— (2000). *Strategic Framework 2001–2003*. Lusaka: Government of the Republic of Zambia, NAC.

Olson, D., and Population Services International (PSI) (2003). Making Abstinence Cool. *AIDSLink:*, (79). Retrieved from www.globalhealth.org/publications/article.php3?id=938

Pilcher, C. D., Tien, H. C., Eron Jr, J. J., Vernazza, P. L., Leu, S. Y., Stewart, P. W., (2004). "Brief but efficient: acute HIV infection and the sexual transmission of HIV." *Journal of Infectious Diseases* 189 (10): 1785–92.

Pinkerton, S. D., and Abramson, P. R. (1997). Effectiveness of condoms in preventing HIV transmission. *Social Science and Medicine, 44*(9), 1303–1312.

Rasing, T. (2003). *HIV/AIDS and Sex Education among the Youth in Zambia: Towards Behavioural Change.* The African Studies Centre. Available at www.ascleiden.nl/pdf/paper09102003.pdf.

Republic of Zambia (2005). *National HIV/AIDS/STI/TB Policy*. Lusaka: Ministry of Health.

Republic of Zambia, and Ministry of Foreign Affairs (2008). "Statement by Mrs. Winnie Natala Chibesakunda, First Secretary, Development Cooperation and International Organizations, Ministry of Foreign Affairs, Zambia on: agenda item 56: advancement of women to the third committee of the 63rd regular session of the United Nations General Assembly." [Electronic Version]. Retrieved October 15, 2008, from www.un.org/womenwatch/daw/documents/ga63/ZAMBIA.pdf.

Saasa, O., and J. Carlsson (1996). *The Aid Relationship in Zambia : a conflict scenario.* Lusaka: Institute for African Studies; Uppsala: Nordic Africa Institute.

Smith, W. (2008). HIV prevention in Zambia: dropping the "C" from ABC. *BETA bulletin of experimental treatments for AIDS : a publication of the San Francisco AIDS foundation, 20*(4), 50.

Solo, J., M. Luhanga, and D. Wohlfahrt (2005). *Repositioning Family Planning—Zambia Case Study: Ready for Change.* New York: The ACQUIRE Project/Engender Health.

Taylor, S. D. (2006). *Culture and Customs of Zambia*. Westport, CT: Greenwood Press.

UNAIDS (2008). *Report on the Global HIV/AIDS Epidemic*. Geneva: UNAIDS

Underwood, C., Hachonda, H., Serlemitsos, E., and Bharath-Kumar, U. (2006). Reducing the risk of HIV transmission among adolescents in Zambia: Psychosocial and behavioral correlates of viewing a risk-reduction media campaign. *Journal of Adolescent Health, 38*(1).

US Agency for International Development (USAID) (2003). "Kaunda campaigns against HIV/AIDS in TV, radio spots." [Electronic Version]. Success Stories: HIV/AIDS. Retrieved October 27, 2010, from www.usaid.gov/our_work/global_health/aids/News/successpdfs/zambiastory4.pdf.

Ustianowski, A. P., S. D. Lawn, and D. N. Lockwood (2006). "Interactions between HIV infection and leprosy: a paradox." *Lancet Infectious Diseases* 6 (6): 350–60.

Walt, G., E. Pavignani, L. Gilson, and K. Buse (1999a). "Health sector development: from aid coordination to resource management." *Health Policy and Planning* 14 (3): 207–18.

— (1999b). "Managing external resources in the health sector: are there lessons for SWAps?" *Health Policy and Planning* 14 (3): 273–84.

Weller, S. C. (1993). "A meta-analysis of condom effectiveness in reducing sexually transmitted HIV." *Social Science and Medicine* 36 (12): 1635–44.

4 HIV/AIDS Education for HIV-Positive Women Living in India

Priya Lall

Introduction

The rapid spread of HIV in developing nations has caused much concern because of its vast implications on socioeconomic development and health on a global scale. India is currently the epicenter of the HIV epidemic in Asia with an estimated 2.5 million patients in 2006 (UNAIDS, 2006), with a third of these cases being women. Ninety-one percent of these women living with HIV/AIDS (WLHA) have been infected by their husband, who typically has been their only sexual partner (UNAIDS and WHO, 2007). These women will be crucial to the future of the epidemic because they act as gatekeepers to their families' healthcare and provide for them financially when the main breadwinner is too unwell to work (D'Cruz, 2002).

However, previous research has illustrated that women's level of HIV awareness in some areas of India can be very low. For example, in one study of pregnant women's acceptance of HIV-related education and counseling in

South India, only a third of respondents knew of the existence of HIV (Samuel et al., 2007). On the other hand, the majority of participants in a similar study conducted in Karnataka by Rogers et al., (2006) had a comprehensive knowledge of sexual modes of transmission of HIV but less than half were aware that it was possible to prevent transmission of HIV from mother to child. This is a cause for concern as experts in the field of HIV/AIDS prevention, such as De Bruyn (2004), have called for better access to voluntary counseling and testing centers for women in developing nations to reduce infant mortality through vertical transmission from mother to child and to improve health outcomes for families. As Firth et al. (2010) stated, "Only with full awareness of the methods of prevention and treatment of HIV will Indian women and their families be able to make appropriate health decisions to protect themselves and their children from this deadly virus."

A set of programs established during the third phase of the National AIDS Control Organization's (NACO) policy enacted in 2006 have attempted to reduce the rate of HIV transmission through public campaigns to increase awareness of HIV in the general population. In addition, coverage of governmental Integrated Counseling and Testing Centers (ICTCs) has been expanded to ensure early detection of HIV in the risk population and increase access to medication for prevention of parent-to-child transmission in pregnant women (Sinha and Roy, 2008). These centers are supposed to follow strict guidelines on provision of HIV testing set by UNAIDS and NACO (2007a), which stipulate that testing should be voluntary, counseling should be offered before and after the test, and the results must be kept confidential unless the patient wishes otherwise. During the pre- and post-test counseling sessions, information provided should include how to prevent further transmission of HIV, which medications should be used to treat HIV, and how the patient can cope with the psychosocial consequences of being HIV-positive.

Previous research on the interaction between patients and their doctors during the testing process illustrates that most of these guidelines are not followed in real life. For instance, Kurien et al. (2007) demonstrated that many doctors in private health-care facilities will test for HIV without their permission patients before invasive surgery. Sheikh and Porter (2010) attributed this behavior to doctors' resistance to medical regulations imposed in a top-down fashion by national organizations such as NACO. They stated: "Doctors conceal their divergent practices, and comply superficially with policies in spite of disagreeing with them, and often fail to engage with the principles of the guidelines they enact." This was because medical practitioners believed that WHO's rights-based approach to dealing with people living with HIV/AIDS (PLWHA) was inappropriate to the Indian cultural context. Consequently, Sheikh and Porter argued that it is "important to enfranchise practitioners' voices and to help them develop the capacity to deliberate appropriate courses of action on the basis of their values and lived experiences."

However, Sheikh and Porter fail to engage with the detrimental impact that failure to follow such guidelines could have on PLWHA's physical and mental health after they are diagnosed with HIV. Datye et al. (2006) explored private practitioners' communication with patients around HIV testing, demonstrating that doctors would adapt their behavior toward their clients according to their perception of their mental health and ability to understand what is being communicated to them. Patients who were uneducated or perceived as having suicidal tendencies were not directly told of their HIV status by their medical practitioner. Among this type of client women and younger patients were seen by doctors as being less capable of understanding a sero-positive diagnosis than other patients. This indicates that health-care practitioners could hold biased attitudes against their female clients, which would make them less inclined to directly inform female clients of their HIV status and provide HIV/AIDS education as part of the diagnosis.

Current research on awareness of HIV and doctor-patient interactions during testing demonstrate that PLWHA face many impediments to receiving appropriate HIV/AIDS education as part of the testing process. These barriers could potentially have a detrimental effect on the physical and psychosocial well-being of WLHA who may have little or no awareness of how to prevent further transmission of the virus or treat their condition. Therefore, this chapter aims to examine which factors impact HIV-positive women's access to HIV/AIDS education during diagnosis.

Methods

This research was conducted in collaboration with four NGOs and three other positive networks (PN), which were located in the districts of Hyderabad, Krishna, West Godavari, and Guntur in Andhra Pradesh (AP). These areas were chosen because they have been identified by NACO as having a prevalence of over 1 percent for more than five years (NACO 2007b). Thirty-three participants were sampled from a population of female HIV-infected patients who are clients of the services at the NGOs and PNs and were approached by the staff at these organizations. These respondents were selected according to Patton's (2002) criteria of "convenience sampling," whereby participants are selected from those willing to undertake interviews, in conjunction with staff in the NGOs and PNs who acted as gatekeepers to the data.

The interview schedule was designed to incur an "illness narrative" from respondents on factors which they believed led to their diagnosis and their experiences of HIV testing. This interview schedule was well paced, with a gentle start before delving into complex questions (Pole and Lampard, 2002). It began with an explanation of the purpose of the research; then the participants were asked "general descriptive" questions (Burgess, 1985), such as age and occupation. The participants were then encouraged to provide their narratives with as little input from the researcher as possible through such questions as "Can you please tell me about your reaction to being diagnosed with HIV?" When the respondents had difficulties answering these questions, they were gently guided into providing their narratives through a set of questions probing into different components of their experience of HIV testing.

Collocation analysis (Mello, 2002) was used to examine the data, whereby the researcher locates the position of the respondents in relation to their narratives through multiple methods. First, narratives within the text were identified by distinguishing their themes and patterns and comparing them with other interview transcripts. These narratives were then coded according to the flow of the story and themes and concepts that recurred within the text. Mathieson and Barrie (1998) effectively used this method of analysis to examine illness narratives of cancer patients by coding sections of their transcript according to the overarching themes of narratives and points of divergence from it.

Results

There were two predominant themes in the respondents' narratives of their HIV testing experiences. The first revolved around "trigger" events that had led to the respondents' diagnosis, such as extreme symptoms of HIV displayed by their spouses. The identification of these types of events was crucial because it influenced the behavior of the practitioner during diagnosis. The second predominant theme was respondent's experience of HIV testing. The narratives illustrated that the doctor's practice of HIV testing was culturally ascribed rather than following an individualistic, rights-based approach as prescribed by governmental agencies.

Trigger events

None of the respondents had, because of a lack of understanding of their risk of HIV, undergone an HIV test; the respondents had either never heard of HIV or had only a rudimentary knowledge of it prior to diagnosis. One participant did not know of the existence of HIV before being diagnosed as sero-positive. She perceived it to be like TB, which does not hold the same type of stigma as HIV does. She said in response to a question of her knowledge of HIV before diagnosis, "[I knew about HIV] not even a pinch. If I heard somebody had died of AIDS, I used to think that is also a disease like TB."

Other respondents who had a low awareness of HIV prior to their diagnosis held stigmatizing views similar to those described in Alonzo and Reynolds's (1995) typology of HIV-related stigma, which took into consideration "'variations in the construction of stigma and strength of negative response." This was achieved by merging dimensions and types of stigma as described by various theorists such as Goffman (1968). One participant who had a low level of knowledge of HIV before diagnosis, most identified with two of the dimensions of stigma highlighted by Alonzo and Reynolds (1995). The first is that HIV is "associated with an undesirable and an unaesthetic form of death." She learned of the existence of HIV after a member of her community died from it. The act of witnessing this neighbor lose copious amounts of weight as her health degenerated convinced her that HIV was a terminal disease. She stated: "I heard of the name when a neighbor of mine died with AIDS. I did not have any knowledge about it . . . I used to get frightened seeing AIDS patients because they would become so thin and ultimately die."

Subsequent to this response, she was asked why she thought her neighbor had died of HIV, to which she answered, "[The neighbor] used to lead a very bad life, having illegal relationships with men and she got the disease and died." This reflects a belief that her neighbor deserved her condition as a product of her sexual behavior. It is possible that she perceived her neighbor's death as *karmic fate* and as a consequence of her leading "a very bad life." This participant's perception of her neighbor aligned with Alonzo and Reynolds's typology of HIV-related stigma as being "tainted by a religious belief as to its immorality and/or thought to be contracted via a morally sanctionable behavior and therefore thought to represent a character blemish." Other respondents described their husband's pre- and extramarital sexual relations in similarly scathing terms, such as "illegal contacts" or as "roaming." Since none of the respondents had indulged in such behavior, they viewed the risk of their contracting HIV before diagnosis as outside the realm of possibility.

Due to their lack of awareness of their risk of potentially contracting HIV, the only factor that led to the HIV testing of the respondents were events that were out of their control and that acted as a trigger to their subsequent diagnosis. There were two types of trigger events that recurred in the respondents' narratives, the first being a routine HIV test as part of antenatal care. Respondents who learned that they were HIV-positive in this manner reported that they underwent the HIV test without much forethought because it was part of standard procedures they undertook as part of antenatal treatment. This could be because these participants perceived the HIV test no differently from many other types of physical examinations, such as urine and blood testing, which they were required to undertake to monitor their health status as part of antenatal treatment (Rani et al., 2008). One participant reported, "Usually when pregnant, we do for all the usual tests, and then they did the HIV test when I came to know that I was HIV positive."

Her narrative encapsulates the thought processes of some WLHA before they undertake a routine HIV test as part of antenatal treatment. She reported that she had willingly undergone the test for reasons that did not encompass her own risk of contracting the virus. She said, "I got myself tested like all other pregnant women and I did not think so deeply and said to myself, 'Why will this disease come to me?'" This illustrates that in her case, the stigma of undertaking a HIV test was mitigated by the fact that it was a common procedure that "other pregnant women" were expected to take. Furthermore, she emphasized that she had no reason to believe that she could possibly be HIV-positive as her only sexual partner had been her husband and thus she had no reason to fear the result. She knew that prior to their marriage, her husband would travel to different areas of India for a period of 2–3 months at a time to sell clothes; during this time he could have been having affairs with other women. However, after they married, he agreed to work in a less mobile occupation as a clerk in a clothes shop, which gave her little reason to suspect that he had extramarital affairs.

The second type of trigger event for many respondents was the admittance of their spouses to a medical facility when they exhibited extreme symptoms of AIDS, such as tuberculosis. There were a few participants whose partner did not have any prior knowledge of their serostatus before they sought treatment. In some of these cases the respondents' spouses were close to death while the respondents themselves had few or no symptoms. This meant that many respondents had little choice but to adopt the burdensome role of their husband's carer. These participants would speak little of their own experience of being diagnosed with HIV and instead described the trauma of witnessing their partner's painful decline from symptoms such as "body pains" and "black complexion" to "stomach motions" and "madness." As most financial resources within the family were diverted toward trying to treat the respondent's spouse, little attention was paid to the need for the respondent and her children to be tested for HIV.

One participant learned that her husband was HIV-positive after he suffered from a fever for a month. *At the time, she attributed this fever to a fight that her husband, an auto-rickshaw driver, had had with a man who drove automobiles and who had "scratched him on his face and eyes." Her husband was diagnosed with typhoid at the first clinic they visited. At the next hospital they visited, they were asked by the practitioners who perhaps suspected the respondent's husband of being sero-positive if an HIV test could be performed. She said,

> We took him to one Suresh Hospital situated at Nakkathota where we incurred a large sum of money up to Rs. 30,000. He had very high fever and they wanted to check his blood which would cost them (her husband's parents) Rs. 1,800 for the specific test. So, we decided to get this test done. It was finally revealed that my husband had HIV.

Her narrative demonstrates the type of obstacle that WLHA may encounter after her partner has been diagnosed as sero-positive and is extremely ill. The most pertinent barrier in this respondent's case was financial, as large sums of money had already been expended on her spouse's treatment before he had been tested for HIV. After her mother-in-law and father-in-law were informed that her husband was HIV-positive, the few financial resources available were used to search for a "cure" for the condition. She was informed by the doctors who treated her husband that she should undertake an HIV test since, as his spouse, she was at risk of contracting HIV. However, she refused, believing that it was more important to concentrate on the needs of her husband as she considered herself healthy enough not to be in need of any type of treatment. She said:

> In spite of the doctors asking me to take the test, I refused. My main concern was that my husband should first get all right and then be able to go about and do his work. At the moment I am quite healthy and I can think of it only later.

Another obstacle to HIV testing was that the physicians did not inform her or her husband of the available types of biomedical treatment for HIV. According to the guidelines on testing and counseling set by NACO, patients diagnosed as HIV-positive should be referred to the nearest health-care facility offering HIV-related treatment. One possible reason for this participant not receiving any information on allopathic treatment of HIV could have been that the doctors had no knowledge of the healthcare available. Datye et al. (2006) reported that many Indian private practitioners had a "lack of knowledge and skills regarding the illness, often [leading to the] referral of patients to HIV 'specialists' who form a select group of practitioners working exclusively with HIV patients." This finding is worrying as previous research on the health-seeking behavior of Indian patients has illustrated that they have a propensity for using private services, which accounts for 87 percent of the total health-care expenditure (Bhatia and Cleland, 2001; Uplekar et al., 1998). Therefore, many PLWHA could at first be diagnosed in a private facility where the practitioner may not have the skills or knowledge to deal with their condition effectively.

Another factor that acted as a barrier to respondents reaching ICTCs was that their husbands concealed their HIV-status for long periods of time, even when they were very unwell. Guidelines on the confidentiality of results, set by NACO in 2007, stipulate that physicians should inform PLWHA's partners of their serostatus with their permission. In the event of the patient's refusal to disclose their HIV status to those at risk of contracting HIV from them, their practitioner is allowed to disclose their test results to the relevant authorities. If this does not have the desired outcome, practitioners can directly inform their patient's sexual partner of their partner's HIV status (NACO 2007a). Before these guidelines were set, it was unclear how this ethical dilemma could be dealt with. One participant believed that her husband knew for a long period of time before his death that he was HIV-positive. She attended the government hospital many times with him when he was being tested for opportunistic infections or undergoing TB treatment. During this time, her husband's doctors and nurses would speak to her about HIV. She commented that when she asked her husband if he was HIV-positive he would deny it. She recalled:

> Doctor told me that he had TB but did not tell me anything else. Later, Doctor spoke to my husband and the nurses used to speak to me about HIV but never told me that my husband had HIV. After his death, when I went to collect his death certificate, they then told me that he had HIV.

Nevertheless, there were a few cases in which the medical practitioners would flout NACO's guidelines on testing and disclosure by directly informing the respondent of their husband's HIV status without seeking his permission first. One respondent's partner attended a private hospital when her partner had a persistent fever three months after they had married. As she did not know of the existence of HIV prior to this episode, she was not sure what condition her husband could be suffering from. Hence, when her husband displayed extreme symptoms of AIDS including fits, she asked the doctors what illness he was suffering from. She stated:

> He was all right for three months after my marriage and then started having fever. I think he had HIV in his system and it was at this stage it started showing out. At that time, I did not know what HIV meant. Till the last moment of his life, we did not know he had HIV. First my in-laws put him into a private hospital. Towards the end of his life, he started getting fits. I then got a doubt and asked the doctor. The doctors asked me what relationship there was between us and the doctor was told that I was his wife. Then, immediately, he said that I too should be tested. It was then revealed that I too had HIV.

Experiences during HIV testing

WLHA who are diagnosed as sero-positive when pregnant require an extensive range of medical services to ensure that HIV is not transmitted vertically from parent to child. The accounts of respondents' experiences of HIV testings while pregnant varied, some receiving no preventative treatment while others were offered a lot of guidance. Their experience was influenced by whether they had been diagnosed before or after the introduction of new policies in 2006 concerning the prevention of parent-to-child transmission. These policies stipulate that all pregnant WLHA should be given a single dose of Nevirapine while in labor, followed by Zidovudine and Lamivudine (3TC) postpartum (Firth et al., 2010). Those who qualify for "first line ART" are also encouraged to undertake elective caesarean surgery to reduce the risk of transmission. WLHA taking such medication to prevent vertical transmission would require clear instruction on how to adhere to the treatment regime and appropriately care for their child.

One participant, who received her diagnosis when pregnant at the age of 13 in 2001, reported that she experienced stigmatizing behavior from medical staff when giving birth and was not informed of measures to prevent vertical transmission of HIV to her child. She commented that the doctors and nurses who attended her during delivery refused to clean her child, told her not to touch the infant, forced her to stay in an "old bed" in the corridor and asked to her to leave early the next day. Therefore, the only person who attended to her needs was her mother who cleaned the floor of blood after she gave birth to her child. She believed that the staff in the hospital behaved toward her in a discriminatory manner because there was little awareness among the general public and medical profession at this time of the modes of HIV transmission. Therefore, they held the stigmatizing assumption that HIV is "contagious and threatening to the community." She stated:

> After the delivery the doctors did not bother about me or my baby. The nurses neither washed my baby on being born and all showed an indifferent attitude to me and the baby. At the time of the delivery, my mother was asked to remove all my clothes and they made her throw away the clothes. No personnel in the hospital touched my belongings . . . When I heard it, I was nerve racked. The public too was not aware of this disease and doctors also looked down on patients suffering with HIV. At that time, we did not know anything about this disease and thought everything was true.

This respondent claimed that she found the whole experience so distressing that it "brought tears to her mind." After she left the hospital, the only instruction she received on her condition was to not breastfeed her child. She never received any preventative treatment during delivery of her child nor was she instructed on how to maintain her own health. It is obvious in her narrative that medical practitioners had so little knowledge of HIV that they had stigmatizing attitudes toward HIV similar to those expressed by respondents who had a low level of awareness prior to their diagnosis. As a consequence, this participant was provided with a poor level of care when pregnant and medical practitioners were unable to provide her with any form of HIV-related education.

In contrast, another respondent reported that she was given psychological support and HIV-related education after being diagnosed with HIV when pregnant in 2007. At the beginning of the counseling session, she was reassured that "many people were suffering with HIV." Hence, she should not be "afraid" of being sero-positive. Those who counseled her probably thought such reassurance would lessen her initial shock at being diagnosed with HIV, but she claimed that she cried when she learned of her HIV status as she was worried that her husband would "scold" her. Then she was told that it would be possible for her to "control" her condition through adherence to ART medication. After this, she was referred to the nearest facility offering treatment to prevent vertical transmission of HIV from parent to child. Two crucial elements made this postdiagnosis guidance possible: first, unlike many of the other respondents' cases, health-care services were available for preventative treatment because this respondent was diagnosed after 2006. Second, her practitioner was fully aware of the modes of HIV transmission and the treatment services available, as she or he may have been tutored in these matters as part of the re-alignment of policy concerning the treatment of PLWHA.

Participants who were diagnosed as sero-positive after their partner exhibited extreme symptoms of AIDS also had diverse experiences of being tested with HIV. Unlike the previous examples, which were the result of recent changes in HIV policy, some participants' experiences were related to dynamics within their family and their relationship to their doctor. This type of experience was most obvious among respondents who were not directly informed of their HIV status by their family doctor, with a few not learning of their serostatus for a long time after their diagnosis. The most striking example of this concerns a respondent who claimed that the local private health-care practitioner conspired with her husband's family to conceal her HIV status from her. This was because her parents-in-law had arranged her marriage to her husband in order to hide his HIV status from the rest of the community, thus enabling his younger siblings to marry. She said, "My husband is the eldest son. Everyone in the home knew about it but used me as their scapegoat to marry him. I knew he had HIV because every test taken was hidden from me."

Her first test for HIV was part of an antenatal treatment procedure. The test results were communicated to the participant's parents-in-law instead of to her. Despite knowing that she was sero-positive, neither her husband nor his family made any attempt to undertake measures to prevent the transmission of HIV to her child. Furthermore, no treatment was offered when she was suffering from "aches, pains, fever" and had "no energy to work" shortly after giving birth. On the other hand, her husband had been using some form of treatment for a long period of time at great expense. She said:

> He [husband] used to pay Rs. 2,000 monthly for medicines but would tell me that he had some pain and stones in the kidney. I used to ask him, "Why are you using medicines?" He was keeping well with the medicines he was taking but I was becoming dark and weak.

This specific narrative illustrates that her husband and his family were willing to use their own resources to ensure their collective well-being. However, they were reluctant to seek health care for the respondent as it could possibly expose her husband's HIV-positive condition. As a consequence of this type of behavior, this respondent was unable to prevent her child from becoming HIV-positive. She said, "If we knew about it earlier, I would have never breastfed my baby and protected her from getting this disease. My life is gone but I would love to protect my little one."

Respondents who were directly informed of their HIV-status by their physician received appropriate post-test counseling. These sessions were designed not only to provide HIV-related education to respondents who were HIV-positive but also to offer them the cognitive tools to psychologically cope with their condition. This was achieved through a process, described by Kleinman (1988), in which the counselor helps the patient to derive meaning from his or her chronic illness by raising "two fundamental questions for the sick person and the social group: Why me? (the question of bafflement) and What can be done? (the question of order and control)" (p. 28). The objective of the early stages of the counseling session was to mitigate against this initial "bafflement" at being diagnosed as sero-positive by informing the patient of various routes by which HIV can be transmitted. One respondent commented that she felt reassured after being told how HIV could be transmitted and that HIV was not infectious and thus would not act as a barrier to her sharing her life with her husband who was also HIV-positive. She said:

> They [the physician] told me that we could get this disease by illegal relationships, injections, transfusions and other than these you cannot get it. Since you both have this disease, you both only can share your life and not with any outsider.

The next stage addresses the "question of order and control" through instruction on the maintenance of the patient's health status and on the type of medication the patient is required to take. During this phase of counseling it was emphasized to respondents that it was not possible to cure their condition, but they could ameliorate symptoms of HIV through adherence to medication, "being clean," and consuming nutritious food. Furthermore, they were informed that it would be necessary for their health status to be continually monitored by their local service provider to ensure that their health was not deteriorating. This illustrated to respondents that their condition could be controlled to such an extent that it could be possible to conduct normal or everyday activities without disablement. One participant said that she was told by her physician, "There are no medicines to completely cure you, but there are medicines which will reduce the potency of the disease. You must come every 15 days for a check up."

The final stage of the counseling consisted of advice on how to mentally cope with being HIV-positive. Respondents were told in vague terms to "be courageous," "not worry," or not to "think bad thoughts." One respondent commented that when she was tested for HIV after her husband had died, she felt that the practitioners were acting in a psychologically supportive manner through their constant reassurance that she should not worry about being sero-positive. She stated:

> They treated us well. They asked me not to get tensed/worried. They also asked me why am I getting tested. I informed them that my husband had recently expired due to HIV, so I am getting tested to know if I am also infected. After I was tested positive they asked me not to worry and start using tablets. They also counseled me.

These narratives illustrate that the purpose of these post-test counseling sessions were not only to provide HIV/AIDS education but also to provide PLWHA with the psychological tools to cope with their condition. Furthermore, respondents were more able to mentally cope with being HIV-positive through advice on available treatments and how to maintain their health status. Such advice emphasizes that HIV is a condition which is not a death-sentence but a chronic illness that is manageable with adherence to medication.

Conclusion

Participants' narratives about their HIV testing experiences illustrate that their access to HIV/AIDS education was a complex and varied process. This was because most respondents had little awareness of HIV prior to diagnosis, with a few not even knowing of the existence of HIV. Moreover, many of the respondents had little reason to believe that it was possible for them to contract HIV as they displayed few sexual risk behaviors, their only lifetime sexual partner being their spouse. The process that led respondents to be tested for HIV were trigger events, such as an HIV test that was a routine part of antenatal treatment or their partner having extreme symptoms of HIV. These trigger events influenced the manner in which they were tested and what type of information they were offered by their physician when they received their diagnosis.

As mentioned earlier, respondents who were diagnosed when pregnant required an HIV/AIDS-related education, which aided them in preventing parent-to-child transmission and enabled them to sufficiently care for their infant. The quality of information that these respondents received was influenced by whether they had been diagnosed before or after the introduction of new policies concerning prevention of parent-to-child transmission in 2006. Those who were diagnosed prior to 2006 did not receive adequate HIV/AIDS-related education as few facilities offered medication to prevent parent-to-child transmission. In contrast, respondents tested after this date were treated appropriately.

Finally, participants who were diagnosed as sero-positive after their partner exhibited extreme symptoms of HIV also had diverse experiences of being tested with HIV. These respondents' experiences were related to dynamics within their family and their relationship to their doctors. There were a few respondents who were not directly informed of their HIV status by their physician.

In conclusion, these narratives illustrate that WLHA's access to HIV/AIDS-related education as part of pre- or post-test counseling is modified by structural and cultural factors. Respondents who had been tested when pregnant were the most affected by structural factors as they needed the relevant medication to prevent their child from becoming infected with HIV during or after birth. Medical practitioners who either did not have the required knowledge of this type of treatment or the necessary medication were unlikely to provide their patients with HIV/AIDS-related education as part of their diagnosis. In contrast, respondents who were tested after their husbands had displayed extreme symptoms of AIDS were more affected by culturally influenced medical practices such as not being directly informed of their HIV status. These cases demonstrate the importance of addressing such practices in order to increase WLHA access to HIV/AIDS-related education during HIV tests.

Questions for reflection

1. What factors impact the access these women have to further education about their illness after learning they are HIV+?
2. What different kinds of stigma did these women experience, and with which people and groups?
3. How did the education levels of medical practitioners impact the experiences of these women?

Reference list

Alonzo, A. A. and N. R. Reynolds (1995). "Stigma, HIV and AIDS: an exploration and elaboration of a stigma trajectory." *Social Science & Medicine* 41 (3): 303–15.

Bhatia, J., and J. Cleland (2001). "Health–care seeking and expenditure by young Indian mothers in the public and private sectors." *Health Policy and Planning* 16 (1): 55–61.

Burgess, R. G. (1985). *Strategies of Educational Research: Qualitative Methods*. London: Philadelphia: Falmer Press.

Datye, V., K. Kielmann, K. Sheikh, D. Deshmukh, S. Deshpande, J. Porter, and S. Rangan. (2006). "Private practitioners' communications with patients around HIV testing in Pune, India." *Health Policy and Planning* 21 (5): 343.

D'Cruz, P. (2002). "Mapping family caregiving variables in HIV/AIDS: a study from Mumbai, India." *International Conference on AIDS, July 7-12, Barcelona, Spain*.

De Bruyn, M. (2004). "Living with HIV: challenges in reproductive health care in South Africa." *African Journal of Reproductive Health*: 8 (1): 92–98.

Firth, J. L. Jeyaseelan, S. Christina, V. Vonbara, V. Jeyaseelan, S. Elan, S. Abraham, I. Joseph, S. David, S. Cu-Uvin, M. Lurie, C. Wanke, and J. Lionel. (2010). "HIV-1 seroprevalence and awareness of mother-to-child transmission issues among women seeking antenatal care in Tamil Nadu, India." *Journal of the International Association of Physicians in AIDS Care (JIAPAC)* 9 (4): 206.

Goffman, E. (1968). *Asylums: Essays on the Social Situation of Mental Patients and other Inmates*. Harmondsworth: Penguin.

Kleinman, A. (1988). *The Illness Narratives: Suffering, Healing and the Human Condition*. New York: Basic Books.

Kurien, M. K. Thomas, R. C. Ahuja, A. Patel, Shyla P. R., N. Wig, M. Mangalani, Sathyanathan, A. Kasthuri, B. Vyas, A. Brojen, T. D. Sudarsanam, A. Chaturvedi, O. C. Abraham, P. Tharyan,

K. G. Selvaraj, and J. Mathew. (2007). "Screening for HIV infection by health professionals in India." *The National Medical Journal of India* 20 (2): 59–66.

Mathieson, C. M., and C. M. Barrie (1998). "Probing the prime narrative: illness, interviewing, and identity." *Qualitative Health Research* 8 (5): 581.

Mello, R. A. (2002). "Collocation analysis: a method for conceptualizing and understanding narrative data." *Qualitative Research* 2 (2): 231.

NACO (2007a). *Guidelines for HIV Testing.* Delhi: NACO.

— (2007b). *Quarterly CMIS Bulletin.* Delhi: NACO.

Patton, M. (2002). *Qualitative Research and Evaluation Methods* (3rd edn). Thousand Oaks, California: Sage.

Pole, C. J., and R. Lampard (2002). *Practical Social Investigation: Qualitative and Quantitative Methods in Social Research.* London: Prentice Hall.

Rani, M., S. Bonu, and S. Harvey (2008). "Differentials in the quality of antenatal care in India." *International Journal for Quality in Health Care* 20 (1): 62–71.

Rogers, A. A. Meundi, A. Amma, A. Rao, P. Shetty, J. Antony, D. Sebastian, P. Shetty, and A. K. Shetty. (2006). "HIV-related knowledge, attitudes, perceived benefits, and risks of HIV testing among pregnant women in rural Southern India." *AIDS Patient Care & STDs* 20 (11): 803–11.

Samuel, N. P. Srijayanth, S. Dharmarajan, J. Bethel, H. Van Hook M. Jacob, V. Junankar, J. Chamberlin, D. Collins, and J. S. Read. (2007). "Acceptance of HIV-1 education and voluntary counselling/ testing by and seroprevalence of HIV-1 among, pregnant women in rural South India." *Indian Journal of Medical Research* 125 (1): 49.

Sheikh, K., and J. D. H. Porter (2010). "Disempowered doctors? A relational view of public health policy implementation in urban India." *Health Policy and Planning* (26) 1: 83–92.

Sinha, A., and M. Roy (2008). "An ICMR task force study of prevention of parent to child transmission (PPTCT) service delivery in India." *52nd All India Annual Conference of IPHA 2008*, January, Delhi, India, p. 200.

UNAIDS and WHO (2006). *AIDS Epidemic Update.* Geneva: UNAIDS and WHO.

— (2007). *ASIA, AIDS Epidemic Update, Regional Summary.* UNAIDS/08.09E/JC1527E. Geneva: UNAIDS and WHO.

Uplekar, M. S. Juvekar, S. Morankar, S. Ranga, and P. Nunn. (1998). "'Tuberculosis patients and practitioners in private clinics in India." *The International Journal of Tuberculosis and Lung Disease : The Official Journal of the International Union Against Tuberculosis and Lung Disease* 2 (4): 324–9.

The Education Sector Response to HIV and AIDS in the Caribbean

5

David James Clarke

Introduction

The Caribbean has the second highest regional HIV prevalence rates in the world after sub-Saharan Africa. While the total number of people infected is relatively modest on a global scale, the impact in small states can be significant, particularly in terms of poverty and human rights. A significant risk lies in the potential impact on the tourism industry, which is a major economic sector in many countries, concerns about which are signaled by the recent HIV impact study on tourism covering five countries (CARICOM, 2009).

The education sector response to HIV in the Caribbean is distinctive and often innovative, offering important lessons for other regions. There is, of course, considerable need for intercountry sharing in the Caribbean itself, as even the larger countries and territories such as Cuba, Jamaica, and Haiti still share many of the characteristics of small states. (Kelly and Bain, 2003). The Caribbean region is complex, including some 30 territories, mostly independent, with about 36 million inhabitants in total. The region is defined and divided politically as much as it is geographically. There is a shared history of slavery, exploitation, and resistance resulting from centuries of British, Dutch, French, and Spanish imperialism. While there is a rather uniformly high level of development across the region, Haiti is still the poorest country in the Americas and is a unique context in terms of HIV/AIDS and education (UNDP, 2010).

HIV in the Caribbean region

Although it accounts for a relatively small share of the global epidemic, the Caribbean, with adult HIV prevalence at about 1.0 percent, has still been more heavily affected by HIV/AIDS than any region outside sub-Saharan Africa (UNAIDS, 2010). The latest evidence suggests that the regional rate of new HIV infections has stabilized with new infections slightly declining over the period 2001–9 (see Table 1). Because data on behavior in the region is sparse, it is difficult to determine whether earlier declines in new infections reflected the natural course of the epidemic or the impact of HIV/AIDS prevention efforts.

Table 5.1. Adult HIV prevalence (15–49)

Country	2002 (%)	2008
Bahamas	3.5	3.0 (1.9%–4.2%)
Barbados	1.2	1.2 (0.8%–1.7%)
Belize	2.0	2.1 (1.2%–3.1%)
Cuba	<0.1	0.1 (0.1%–0.2%)
Dominican Republic	2.5	1.1 (0.9%–1.2%)
Guyana	2.7	2.5 (1.4%–3.7%)
Haiti	6.1	2.2 (1.9%–2.5%)
Jamaica	1.2	1.6 (1.1%–2.1%)
Trinidad and Tobago	2.5	1.5 (1%–2.1%)

Source: UNAIDS (2010).

The Caribbean region has a mixture of generalized and concentrated epidemics. The national HIV/AIDS burden varies considerably within the region, ranging from an extremely low HIV prevalence in Cuba to 3 percent among adults in the Bahamas. Overall there are only about 240,000 people living with HIV, a relatively low number that has remained stable since the late 1990s. Trying to generalize the entire region by average prevalence or incidence incurs the same problems as doing so for a large country: national data tend to obscure local epidemics and substantial differences in the HIV burden. There is a nearly sevenfold variation in HIV prevalence between the different regions of the Dominican Republic, with especially high rates in and near sugar plantations. This lack of consistence also makes data collection difficult when the use of prevalence numbers from one area can possibly distort the situation. In Haiti, for instance, HIV prevalence among pregnant women in 2006–7 ranged from 0.75 percent in a sentinel antenatal site in the western part of the country to 11.75 percent in one urban setting.

Unprotected sex between men and women, especially paid sex, is the main mode of HIV transmission in the region. Commercial sex is not restricted to women and men are not the only clients (Allen, 2002). Neither is all transmission through heterosexual sex only. A mapping of men who have sex with men (MSM) in Jamaica found this population to be large and heterogeneous (Royes, 2003). Bisexuality was denied and denigrated both by the MSM population and by heterosexuals, but it was directly and indirectly present in the results of the study. Verbal and physical abuse from the police, the outside community, and by their own men is a concern for MSM. This makes life and relationships vulnerable and fragile and negates any intentions for long-term or safe relationships. It also makes it important for researchers and policy makers to be careful about terminology and data collection tools when dealing with different identities versus sexual behaviors in this region. Consequently, education then serves as a tool not only to promote condom use and frequent HIV and STD testing, but also to reduce stigma about different sexualities and the human rights of commercial sex workers and those who have homosexual relationships.

The Caribbean remains the only region, besides sub-Saharan Africa, where women and girls outnumber men and boys among people living with HIV. Women account for approximately half of all infections, with prevalence especially high among adolescent and young women who tend to have infection rates significantly higher than males their own age. High infection levels have been found among female sex workers, including 4 percent in the Dominican Republic, 9 percent in Jamaica, and 27 percent in Guyana.

The high level of population mobility in the Caribbean makes this epidemic complex (Borland et al., 2004). With the movement of groups of people and individuals, there are also often high-risk behaviors that lead to greater vulnerability to HIV infection. It is important to note that the largest movement of people in the Caribbean is generated by recreational visitors to the region. Unsurprisingly, there is some evidence that tourism and HIV are related in the Caribbean, though this is sensitive for governments and under-researched. Some have argued that wealthy tourists, on vacation and relatively more anonymous than in their home country, indulge in riskier sexual behaviors, especially in paying for sex and having multiple partners. Tourism-dependent economies have some of the highest HIV prevalence rates and the available research shows that there is a wide range of arrangements that exist between the tourist and sex worker (PANCAP, 2009). The region has a long historical legacy of sexual exploitation (Grenade, 2007). Marginalized and disadvantaged women and men are implicated in the patterns of "structural violence" that shape the HIV epidemic; sex workers with few life opportunities and resources make a way for themselves in an unequal world (Brennan, 2004; Padilla, 2007).

Finally, there is the universal problem of HIV-related stigma and discrimination. Because of such stigma, the rights of people living with HIV and their families are often violated in the region, simply because they are known or presumed to have HIV/AIDS (Aggleton et al., 2003). This violation of rights increases the negative impact of the epidemic at many levels. In the education sector, cases of children living with HIV being barred from school have been recorded in the region. Stigma attached to taboo sexualities or behaviors such as men having sex with men or transactional sex become linked to HIV/AIDS, as many assume this is the only way infection occurs. Entire populations of people, linked by perceptions about their sexualities or behaviors and moralities, are then linked to the disease, and it is not uncommon for people who do not identify with these groups to engage in risky sexual behaviors because they feel "safe." Stigma, in the Caribbean context, is cyclical.

Youth and HIV in the Caribbean

While the population of the Caribbean is culturally diverse, among youth (10–24 years of age) there are a handful of commonalities. The

World Bank (2003) has identified the following trends among youth in the region:

- Sexual and physical abuse is high and socially accepted in many countries.
- The onset of sexual initiation outside marriage is the earliest in the world.
- The incidence of rage among young people is extremely high and the proportion of adolescent males who carry firearms is extremely high.
- Youth unemployment is especially high in some countries (e.g. St. Lucia, Dominica, St. Vincent and the Grenadines, and Jamaica).
- There is widespread acceptance of alcohol and marijuana in some countries.
- The costs of risky adolescent behavior are high and include teen pregnancy, crime, school drop-out, and HIV.

The situation of children and adolescents involved in prostitution should be given special and separate consideration since their needs and realities are frequently different from those of adults. Pathways leading to high-risk behaviors and sex work of all types must be better understood and should be addressed earlier rather than later in their lives. The lack of real development strategies that include the majority of the population of countries and the poor in particular is acknowledged to be a serious problem in the region (PANCAP, 2009). Governments need to pay more attention to linking education with the world of work. More technical and vocational education and training programs are needed, especially for women and youth.

Behavioral surveillance surveys (BSS) provide useful strategic information for HIV prevention among youth both in and out of school. BSS undertaken in six countries of the Organization of the Eastern Caribbean States (OECS) found that many youth in school did not know the basics of HIV prevention and still believed in common myths (CAREC, et al., 2007). Because the majority reported that they were still virgins, it was concluded that the potential exists for promoting delayed sexual debut as well as empowerment around safer sex before these children become sexually active. It was recommended that HIV prevention be embedded in broader sexual health initiatives as well as fostering greater involvement of people living with HIV in prevention and antistigma activities. In Guyana, the BSS findings showed that out-of-school youth were better able to identify three ways of preventing HIV than those in school (Ministry of Health et al., 2004). Among the latter group, almost half of the males (43 percent) were sexually experienced and 24 percent reported involvement in transactional sex.

A number of country studies have been carried out in the area of adolescent development and rights. The studies conducted in Jamaica, for example, include a strong focus on sexuality and the factors that shape early initiation of sexual activity (UNICEF and UNFPA, 2002). Studies such as these potentially provide value information for HIV education programming, including curriculum content, but it is unclear to what extent this information is being utilized.

Key challenges

These culturally diverse small states pose distinctive challenges for the education sector in responding to HIV/AIDS. Mobilizing the education sector within the multisectoral response to HIV/AIDS has been a consistent challenge across the region since it was first recognized that HIV/AIDS is an education issue. Each state's ministry of education must understand its role in HIV prevention as well as the impact of HIV/AIDS on education and society in general (Kelly, 2000). This includes education aimed at reducing HIV-related stigma and discrimination. There has to be a comprehensive and systemic approach to the education response involving integration in sector policies, plans, core curriculum, preteacher training and in-service teacher training as well as supervision and support at school, in classroom teaching and cocurricular activities and assessment practices (UNESCO and EDC, 2005).

Developing strategies that factor in the particular education issues of small states is another challenge this region faces. There needs to be recognition of the particular strengths and challenges that small states face in developing and sustaining an appropriate education-sector response to HIV. Education development in small states was an important area of research in the 1980s, but this has been somewhat marginalized by the increased focus on large states by development agencies. Nevertheless, the issues identified by Bray (1992) remain pertinent. These include the development of technical capacity in small bureaucracies where staff often perform multiple functions, have access to specialist skills and resources, recognize their vulnerability to the loss of key staff, and finally, lack economies of scale to justify investment in new interventions. In addition, there are issues of economic, political, and environmental vulnerability (Charles et al., 1997)

Small states such as those of the Caribbean region also have potential advantages. Scaling-up should be theoretically less problematic than in larger countries; data, easier to obtain and manage; and implementation problems, easier to diagnose and address. With the strong interpersonal networks characteristic of small states, community participation ought to be more successful. Ongoing improvements in communication technology and transportation should also reduce the isolation of small states and facilitate regional cooperation. Strategies for small states to develop education responses to HIV/AIDS need to ensure that regional cooperation provides economies of scale and scarce technical skills to support sustainable capacity building in the ministries of education and the strengths of the communities are harnessed to support school-based efforts.

Developing and implementing effective and efficient HIV education programs is the most obvious challenge to the education response. There is increasing international research to inform national HIV policy development and programming. Responding to the national HIV/AIDS epidemic requires "knowing the epidemic," or understanding the contextual the factors that drive HIV transmission to ensure that the education response truly matches the epidemic (UNAIDS, 2007) Arguably, the most influential contribution to understanding what makes for effective school-based HIV education has come from Kirby et al. (2006) and his identification of 17 success-factor characteristics. These have been refined and included in UNESCO's recently published guidelines on sexuality education (UNESCO, 2009). The key areas which have been identified concern curriculum development, content, teaching methods, and implementation. Clarke (2008) has highlighted the critical importance of teachers, their engagement and activism in HIV issues, training, and ongoing support in the delivery of effective HIV education.

Finally, building sustainable capacity in HIV education is a major challenge, with the World Bank and UNESCO advocating for a framework for the education sector response. Endorsed by the Council for Human and Social Development (COHSOD) of the Caribbean Community (CARICOM) in 2006, it includes frameworks on sector policy, planning and management, prevention, and a framework especially for HIV/AIDS-related orphans and vulnerable children. The Caribbean region is unusually advanced in terms of guidance and toolkits for education and HIV/AIDS. In 2004, the International Labour Organization (ILO) and UNESCO launched an initiative to draft a model education sector workplace policy for the region based on the *Code of Practice on HIV/AIDS and the World of Work* (ILO, 2001). Regional guidelines for education policy development on HIV have been prepared (Clarke. D, 2008) as well as a toolkit for involving NGOs effectively in the response (Pulizzi et al., 2009). A toolkit has also recently been developed by UNESCO to promote the "Greater Involvement of People living with HIV/AIDS" (or, the "GIPA principle") in the education sector (UNESCO and EDC, 2010). A monitoring and evaluation framework for a comprehensive HIV response has recently been developed for the region as well as a capacity-building toolkit to support its implementation (EDC and UNESCO, 2010a, 2010b).

There are gaps in the guidance available. Perhaps the largest of these is the absence of evidence-based guidance on how to ensure that education sector plans adequately include the HIV response. Another key issue is ensuring that regional guidance is used effectively and translated into national action. As many of these tools are quite recent developments, it is too early to make causal claims about any impact.

The education response to HIV and AIDS

The education sector response to HIV/AIDS in the Caribbean is relatively well documented. Studies on the response in Commonwealth countries of the region agree that it was slow to begin and the national response focused mainly on the health sector (Kelly and Bain, 2003). In the case of Cuba, the provision of free and universal health care has successfully contributed to limiting the spread of HIV along with strong civil-society participation in health and a tradition of intersectoral government (Abreu et al., 2006). Barbados also has had a successful health sector response which is recognized to be due in part to long-term achievements in education which can be traced back to the provision of free secondary education in the 1960s. In effect, education has provided the essential basis for improvement in health and helped to ensure that sufficient expertise was available to address HIV when it emerged (Walrond and Roach, 2006).

During the 1980s and 1990s, HIV education was a small element in the regional Health and Family Life (HFLE) curriculum, targeted at lower secondary education in grades 7–9. Prior to 2002, there was little to show at the school level. The teacher-training curriculum had not been changed to address HIV in HFLE and no teaching materials had been published for it (Morrissey, 2005). Ministries of education were slow to develop policy and strategies for HIV education (CARICOM, 2009). Among the reasons identified were a lack of sustained political will, lack of broad-based stakeholder involvement and ownership, multiple and overloaded curricula and poor vision and strategic planning. Countries in the Caribbean region are now strengthening their School Health and Nutrition (SHN) capacity with external support from UN agencies, the World Bank, NGOs, and the private sector.

Mobilizing the education sector within the multisectoral response

Good progress is being made in mobilizing the education sector response within the national response framework. A litmus test for the inclusion of the education sector in the national response to HIV is the extent to which countries report on life skills education and orphan school attendance indicators (11 and 12) within country reports on progress related to the 2001 UNGASS Declaration of Commitment on HIV and AIDS. UNGASS country reporting, which happens every two years, is in fact the *only* international reporting framework that includes the education sector response to HIV/AIDS. Reporting on Education for All (EFA), in contrast, has conspicuously failed in successive Global Monitoring Reports (GMRs) to develop an agreed set of indicators for life skills/HIV education and use them. The UNGASS indicator (11) on life skills education is primarily one of coverage or access. It aims to measure the percentage of schools that provided life-skills-based HIV education within the last academic year. Almost all countries that have submitted UNGASS Country reports for 2010 include data on indicator 11 (see Table 2). It is helpful to disaggregate the response by level of education, that is, by primary and secondary education. Some countries, for example, Barbados, Cuba, and Grenada now do this. Many countries also include a narrative and additional data on life-skills education in their UNGASS reports.

There is widest possible range of performance in life-skills education coverage from 0 percent (Suriname) to 100 percent (Barbados, Cuba, Grenada, Guyana, and St. Vincent and the Grenadines). High levels of coverage are also reported in Antigua and Barbuda, and the Bahamas. Low levels are reported in the Dominican Republic and Haiti. A number of countries still have a long way to achieve 100 percent coverage. A number of countries are implementing programs at both primary and secondary levels.

Table 5.2. UNGASS on HIV and AIDS indicators

Country	Life-skills coverage (Indicator 11)	Orphan school attendance (Indicator 12)	HIV Knowledge among 15–24 year olds (Indicator 13)
Antigua and Barbuda	85%	All education is free and compulsory	48%
Bahamas	77.63%	100%	No data available
Barbados	100% (secondary) 80.6% (primary)	All education is free and compulsory	50.43% (51.9% male: 48.9% female)
Belize	46.5% (primary)	62% (double orphan) 93.6% (single orphan)	50.2%
Cuba	100% (secondary) 70.9% (primary)	100%	58.4%
Dominican Republic	6.16%	69.23 % (double orphan) 97.09 % (single orphan)	40.8% (female) 37.32 (male)
Grenada	75% (secondary) 100% (primary)	No data available	No data available
Guyana	23.8 % (secondary) 73.9 % (primary)	No data available	45%
Haiti	12.6%	86%	40.4% (male) 31.9% (female)
Jamaica	44%	0.99	37.4% (male) 42.3% (female)
St. Kitts and Nevis	45%	Data not relevant	52%
St. Lucia	59%	100%	59%
St. Vincent and the Grenadines	100%	No data available	49% (59% male: 40% female 15–19 years)
Suriname	0%	No data available	41%
Trinidad and Tobago	No data available	No data available	No data available

Attention to school attendance by orphans has received less attention (Indicator 12). A number of countries present no data or assume that because there is free and compulsory education, there is no problem. This may indeed be the case, but it is apparent from those countries which provide data there is a problem in retaining double orphans in school (i.e. children who have lost both parents).

UNGASS country reporting offers a mechanism for periodic stock taking at a regional level. Other potential indicators of sector mobilization such as HIV policy and strategic plan development in the sector are discussed below in the section on sustainable capacity.

Developing strategies which factor in the particular education issues of small states

We have seen earlier that regional organizations have been proactive in developing guidelines and tools to assist country-level activity. The regional response has provided small states with technical assistance and frameworks for development of the education sector response to HIV, though it was slow to develop. The CARICOM Regional Framework Strategic Plan for HIV and AIDS 2002–6 did not specifically address the education sector (World Bank, 2008). Steps were put in place in 2006 for capacity building at the regional level and technical assistance at the country level while a network of Caribbean education sector HIV coordinators was established (EDUCAN) with annual meetings planned to support capacity building in key areas such as monitoring and evaluation.

The curriculum for HIV prevention is a regional endeavor. Health and Family Life Education (HFLE) is an initiative of the Caribbean Community (CARICOM), which comprises 14 Member States and 5 Associate Members. HFLE has a long history, introduced into the formal curriculum in the mid-1960s as Family Life Education and since then has significantly evolved (Rampersad, 2010). In 1996, ministers of education and health endorsed the key document, *A Strategy for Strengthening Health and Family Life Education (HFLE) in CARICOM Member States*.

The Council for Human and Social Development (COHSOD) in 2003 endorsed the need to develop a Life-Skills-based HFLE Regional Curriculum Framework. This framework, with regional standards and core outcomes, shifted the focus from what was a knowledge-based curriculum to one that would be life-skills based. This framework was intended to serve as a guide to member states to review or develop their national life-skills HFLE curriculum. Additionally, COHSOD agreed that HFLE should be a core area of instruction at all levels of the education, and should also be used to develop out-of-school youth programs.

The Regional Framework for HFLE was developed for children aged 9–14 years; the Core Curriculum Guide for Teachers was revised, and teachers, teacher educators, curriculum officers and HFLE coordinators were identified from all levels of the education system and trained as trainers in life-skills education.

HFLE is the carrier for the main regional response to HIV prevention education. It is a curriculum initiative that not only reinforces the connection between health and education, but also uses a holistic approach within a planned and coordinated framework. It is a comprehensive, life-skills-based program, which focuses on the development of the whole person (Constantine, 2006). It aims to:

- Enhance the potential of young persons to become productive and contributing adults/citizens;
- Promote an understanding of the principles that underlie personal and social well-being;
- Foster the development of knowledge, skills, and attitudes that make for healthy family life;
- Provide opportunities to demonstrate sound health-related knowledge, attitudes, and practices;
- Increase the ability to practice responsible decision making about social and sexual behavior; and
- Aim to increase the awareness of children and youth of the fact that the choices they make in everyday life profoundly influence their health and personal development into adulthood.

The content for HFLE is organized around four themes: sexuality and sexual health; self and interpersonal relationships; eating and fitness; and managing the environment. Standards and core outcomes have been developed for each theme. The effectiveness of HFLE in delivering HIV learning outcomes has not yet been adequately evaluated, and the broad-ranging program offers sex education as just one of many components, though it does discuss high-risk behaviors such as MSM and transactional sex.

Multiple barriers to effective HFLE provision at school level have been identified. They include insufficient teacher training, lack of teacher confidence in delivering HFLE, perceived community resistance, lack of time and resources and social taboos regarding sexuality education content. The subject is not compulsory and assessing outcomes is problematic because students are not tested on the curriculum. As a result, HFLE lacks "legitimate" status in the curriculum (Plummer, 2010).

The relatively low levels of HIV knowledge presented in Table 2 (Indicator 13) indicate that HFLE is not yet working adequately. The HFLE baseline study undertaken in Jamaica with JICA support found a wide range in the number of hours being allocated to HFLE in schools (Ministry of Education,

2008). However, a high level (80 percent) of guidance counselors who teach the subject reported they felt comfortable in teaching about sexuality. The main problems related to the lack of resource materials and trained personnel. It was also found that life skills education methods were not widely known by teachers.

In September 2005, a three-year study involving implementation, monitoring, and evaluation of an HFLE curriculum based on the regional framework was begun in four pilot countries: St. Lucia, Barbados, Grenada, and Antigua. The curriculum covered two themes: sexuality and sexual health (including HIV prevention), and self and interpersonal relationships (including violence prevention). The study involved both process and impact evaluation methodologies (UNICEF, 2009). The process evaluation revealed the following:

- Teachers were overall very enthusiastic about the curriculum and most were comfortable with the content.
- Lessons were judged to be developmentally and culturally appropriate.
- The topics were considered to be important.
- Nearly 60 percent of intervention school teachers reported the importance of HFLE but less than 20 percent did so in comparison schools.
- Teachers were concerned that there was insufficient time to complete lesson material and had ongoing problems scheduling HFLE class time.
- Many teachers had little classroom experience including using the interactive pedagogic strategies in HFLE.
- Substantial teacher turnover impeded lesson completion and late teacher assignments made planning for training difficult.

The impact evaluation data reveal no pattern of significant positive effects of the HFLE curriculum on the self-reported attitudes, behaviors and skills in health domains relating to the themes of self and interpersonal relationships, and sexuality and sexual health of Form 3 students. While there were no significant negative effects either, this is perhaps scant consolation.

A regional success story for HIV prevention education appears to be the Programa de Educacion Afectivo Sexual (PEAS) or Sex Education Program (Beasley et al., 2008). The program is integrated into the core secondary school curriculum and covers prevention and transmission of STIs, including HIV and the promotion of gender equality and human rights with a view to strengthening the capacity of students to make conscious and responsible decisions concerning sexual behaviors. PEAS also includes a peer education component aimed at providing peer support and counseling involving parents and caregivers while supporting community action and outreach for health change. Such involvement, however, has been varied across schools.

The active support of religious authorities has been an important success factor. The program is managed by each school's counseling and psychology unit and employs a holistic approach to support students in skills building and values acquisition. The school principal is ultimately responsible for ensuring the PEAS curriculum is implemented. All teachers are provided with a set of grade-appropriate materials which include two main manuals. Teenagers were involved in the materials development process. The materials are used in teacher training and classroom teaching. Supplementary resources including from the Ministry of Health are used to inform and support teaching.

Implementation of PEAS has revealed a number of challenges and lessons learned. Teachers identified the need to strengthen training and provide adequate support during program implementation. Introduction of the peer education component is increasing student participation and sense of ownership of the program but greater efforts are needed to put in place a mechanism to improve the participation of parents in the program and actively contribute to the achievement of its objectives. A strategic action plan exists, but regional and district level action plans are also required as well as school-based work plans and lesson plans. Finally, there is a need for a monitoring and evaluation framework to track both process and outcomes.

Building sustainable capacity in HIV education

A preliminary assessment of ministry of education (MoE) capacity was undertaken by EDC in 2006, and found that only two countries, Jamaica and Haiti, had developed a specific HIV policy and only in Jamaica was it being implemented (Whitman and Oomen, 2010). The cabinet in Jamaica approved HIV Policy for the Jamaican Ministry of Education in 2004. This was the first in the region. However, 13 countries had developed policies for HFLE, 12 of which were based on the regional framework. Thirteen countries had trained teachers in HFLE, while eight of these had trained teachers specifically in HIV education. Six MoEs were providing access to services such as counseling and VTC and nine MoEs had made efforts to involve PLWHA , though these were not judged to be very effective. Eight MoEs were implementing programs to address the needs of OVCs. Most MoEs were partnering with NGOs to provide services for OVCs and youth.

A rapid survey was more recently undertaken by EDUCAN with support from ECD, PCD, the World Bank and UNESCO (O'Connell et al., 2009). The findings reveal that progress has taken place across the region, but that much remains to be done. Five countries now have education sector policies on HIV including workplace issues. Four countries have policies on SHN (Barbados, Guyana, St. Kitts and Nevis, and Trinidad and Tobago). In Barbados and Guyana, SHN policy is implemented jointly by the ministries of education and health. In St. Kitts and Nevis, and Trinidad and Tobago, it is the responsibility of the ministry of health.

While all 13 countries, with the exception of Anguilla, reported that they had put in place national HIV strategies, only six had education-sector strategies (Barbados, Belize, Grenada, Guyana, Jamaica, and St. Vincent and the Grenadines). Only four countries have both an education strategy and an HIV strategy for the sector (Barbados, Grenada, Guyana, and Jamaica).

The most detailed HIV plan for the education sector appears to be that of Jamaica for the period 2007–12 (Ministry of Education, 2008). Jamaica was the first country in the region to undertake a comprehensive situation and response analysis of the education-sector response to HIV, with support from UNESCO (Clarke, 2008. This process informed the implementation of HIV interventions of the Jamaican Ministry of Education and Youth (MoEY) and supported the development of a strategic plan. The policy is a living document and was revised in 2010.

Six countries have a unit for SHN in their ministries of education (Anguilla, Barbados, Guyana, Jamaica, St. Vincent and the Grenadines, and Trinidad and Tobago), and three have HIV units (Antigua, Bahamas, and Jamaica). Full-time HIV coordinators are to be found in all of the above, except Anguilla. Countries with neither SHN nor HIV Units are: Belize, Dominica, St. Lucia, and St. Kitts and Nevis.

All countries, except Anguilla, report that teachers are trained in life-skills education. Only four do this in preservice teacher education (Antigua, Belize, Guyana, and St. Vincent and the Grenadines). The rest rely on in-service teacher training, which is also used by those implementing it in preservice training. Seven countries report that SHN training is given in preservice training (Antigua, Bahamas, Belize, Grenada, Guyana, St. Vincent and the Grenadines, and Trinidad and Tobago). All countries report that HIV training is given in in-service teacher training.

Jamaica has established the HIV/AIDS Response Team (HART), an innovative mechanism which operates at both central and decentralized levels of the education system. There are two officers in each region. This provides a vehicle for capacity building, policy dissemination as well as monitoring and evaluation. Health Advisory Committees are required to be set up in all schools and learning institutions.

Ten countries report that HIV prevention education is delivered through nonformal education (Antigua, Dominica, and Grenada do not do this); five of these NFE approaches use a life-skills-based approach. Peer education is used in all of these. HIV education in NFE appears to be a neglected area of education sector development. Peer education is also used in secondary schools in 11 of the countries (Anguilla and Antigua do not take this approach). It is used in primary schools in three countries (Guyana, St. Kitts and Nevis, and St. Lucia).

Conclusions

This chapter has covered the overall educational response to HIV/AIDS in the Caribbean. While generalities can be made, analyzing the policy response of different countries and even agencies is often more useful. The social, economic and cultural context of this region also must be taken into account when reviewing the education response. So far, the international community has learned specific lessons from the Caribbean education response.

- Country-level UNGASS reporting provides a good and improving window on the education sector response in the region.
- The regional response to HIV in the education sector has added significant value to what can be achieved by small countries individually, but in the final analysis, national commitment by government and civil society is critical to success.
- The impressive array of regional tools and guidelines needs to be reviewed regularly to ensure it is fit for purpose.
- Coverage of HIV education is increasing or at high levels in many countries, but program effectiveness is in question.
- The main framework for HIV education, HFLE, is not yet proven to be effective. Numerous constraints to implementation exist and HFLE does not meet all of the identified characteristics of effective programs. The core curriculum lacks a clear focus on high-risk behaviors and their prevention; sexuality is just one of several components.

- There is also a need to generate localized teaching and learning materials, given the diversity of cultures and HIV epidemics in the region.
- Preservice teacher education, particularly for life-skills methods, needs to be strengthened.
- Access to youth-friendly health services also needs to be strengthened.
- HFLE needs to be kept under regular review with a strong focus on assessing process indicators and learning outcomes in relation to sexuality and HIV education.
- Sustainable capacity building is a work in progress across the region. Countries are increasingly putting in place policies and plans for HIV education within a broader SHN framework. More attention is required to embed HIV programming in mainstream education sector planning and to plan systematically for capacity building in sexuality and HIV education;
- The education response to HIV in Jamaica is particularly innovative, a result of MoE commitment and well-targeted development assistance. The PEAS sex-education program in the Dominican Republic has many noteworthy features, not least the explicit focus on sexuality education.
- Haiti requires a separate approach and additional resources, given the status of its education system.

These lessons are important to consider not just for the Caribbean context, but especially for small states with similar histories worldwide. Country-specific lessons can also be generalized to fit similar situations, and as a reminder of the uniqueness of each epidemic.

Questions for reflection

1. How have policy-makers considered both local and regional aspects of this epidemic in the Caribbean?
2. How can small states work with regional organizations to strengthen their educational response?
3. What are the similarities and differences between regions like the Caribbean and large, diverse countries such as the United States of America or India in terms of HIV/AIDS education policy?

Reference list

Abreu , M., J. Waller, J. J. J. Fiol, J. P. Avila, R. T. Peña, M. S. Peña, R. O. Soto, and G. E. Torres. (2006). "Cuba." In Beck, E., N. Mays, A. W. Whiteside, and J. M. Zunig (eds), *The hiv Pandemic: Local and Global Implications*. Oxford: Oxford University Press.

Aggleton, P., R. Parker, and M. Maluwa. (2003). *Stigma, Discrimination and hiv/aids in Latin America and the Caribbean*. Technical Working Papers Series. Washington, DC: Sustainable Development Department, Inter-American Development Bank.

Allen, C. (2002). "Gender and Transmission of HIV in the Caribbean." Annual Conference Papers, vol. 3, ed. S. Courtman. London: The Society for Caribbean Studies.

Beasley, M., A.Valerio and D. A. P. Bundy (eds). (2008). *A Sourcebook of hiv/aids Prevention Programs*. Volume 2, *Education Sector-Wide Approaches*. Washington, DC: World Bank.

Borland, R., R. Borland, L. Faas, D. Marshall, R. McLean, M. Schroen, M. Smit, and T. Valerio. (2004). *HIV/AIDS and Mobile Populations in the Caribbean: A Baseline Assessment*. Santo Domingo: IoM.

Bray, M. (1992). *Educational Planning in Small Countries*. Paris: UNESCO.

Brennan, D. (2004). *What's Love Got to Do with It? Transnational Desires and Sex Tourism in the Dominican Republic*. Durham: Duke University Press.

CAREC (2007). *Behavioural surveillance surveys in six countries of the Organization of Eastern Caribbean States*, 2005–2006. March. Port of Spain.

Charles, E. (1997). *A Future for Small States: Overcoming Vulnerability*. London: Commonwealth Secretariat.

Clarke, D. (2008). *Heroes and Villains: Teachers in the Education Response to HIV*. Paris: International Institute for Educational Planning, UNESCO.

Constantine, C. (2006). *Health and Family Life Education: Teacher Training Manual*. Newton, MA: EDC.

EDC and UNESCO (2010a). *Monitoring and Evaluation Framework for a Comprehensive HIV and AIDS Response in the Caribbean Education Sector*. Kingston, Jamaica: UNESCO and Newton, MA: EDC.

— (2010b). *Capacity Building Toolkit for Monitoring and Evaluating a Comprehensive HIV and AIDS Response in the Caribbean Education Sector*. Kingston, Jamaica: UNESCO and Newton, MA: EDC.

Grenade, W. (2007). "Crisis, chaos and change: Caribbean development challenges in the twenty-first century." Paper presented at the SALISES 8th Annual Conference, Trinidad and Tobago, March 26–8.

HEU Centre for Health Economics, Faculty of Social Sciences, The University of the West Indies, Trinidad and Tobago. (2009). *HIV and Tourism Study: Slow Onset Disasters and Tourism Development: Exploring the Economic Impact of HIV/AIDS on the Tourism Industry in Selected Caribbean Destinations*. Georgetown, Guyana: CARICOM Secretariat and Pan Caribbean Partnership against HIV/AIDS (PANCAP).

ILO (2001). *An ilo Code of Practice on hiv/aids and the World of Work*. Geneva: ILO.

Kelly, M. J. (2000). *Planning for Education in the Context of hiv/aids: Fundamentals of Educational Planning No: 66*. Paris: International Institute for Educational Planning, UNESCO.

Kelly, M., and B. Bain (2003). *Education and HIV/AIDS in the Caribbean*. Kingston: Ian Randle Publishers.

Kirby, D., A. Obasi, and B.A. Laris. (2006). The effectiveness of sex education and HIV education interventions in schools in developing countries. In Ross, D. A. David, B. Dick, and J. Ferguson, (eds), *Preventing hiv/aids in Young People: a Systematic Review of the Evidence from Developing Countries*. Geneva: WHO.

Ministry of Education (2008). *Health and Family Life Education (HFLE) Baseline Survey: Preliminary Report.* Kingston, Jamaica: MoE and JICA.

Ministry of Health, USAID, and FHI (2004). *Behavioural Surveillance Survey.* Georgetown, Guyana: Ministry of Health, USAID, and FHI .

Morrissey, M. (2005*). Response of the Education Sector in the Commonwealth Caribbean to the HIV/ AIDS Epidemic.* Kingston, Jamaica: ILO.

Padilla, M. (2007). *Caribbean Pleasure Industry: Tourism, Sexuality and AIDS in the Dominican Republic.* Chicago, IL: University of Chicago Press.

PANCAP (2009). *Prostitution, Sex Work and Transactional Sex in the English, Dutch and French Speaking Caribbean: A Literature Review of Definitions, Laws and Research.* Georgetown, Guyana: CARICOM.

Plummer. D. (2010). "HIV in Caribbean schools: the role of HIV education in the second most severely affected region in the world." In M. Morrissey, M. Bernard, and D. Bundy (eds), *Challenging hiv and aids: A New Role for Caribbean Education.* Kingston, Jamaica: UNESCO.

Pulizzi, S., P. Russell-Brown, D. Clarke, C. Constantine, and L. Rosenblum. (2009). *Ensuring Quality: Ministry of Education and Ngos Responding to the AIDS Pandemic.* Newton, MA: EDC.

Rampersad, J. (2010). "Health and family life education in the formal education sector in the Caribbean: a historical perspective." In M. Morrissey, M. Bernard, and D. Bundy (eds), *Challenging HIV and AIDS: A New Role for Caribbean Education.* Kingston, Jamaica: UNESCO.

Royes, H. (2003). *HIV/AIDS Risk Mapping of Men Who Have Sex with Men in Jamaica.* Jamaica HIV/ AIDS Prevention and Control Project. Kingston, Jamaica: Ministry of Health.

UNAIDS (2007). *Practical Guidelines for Intensifying HIV Prevention: Towards Universal Access.* Geneva: UNAIDS.

——— (2010). *Global Report: UNAIDS Report on the Global AIDS Epidemic, 2010.* Geneva: UNAIDS.

UNDP (2010). *The Real Wealth of Nations: Pathways to Human Development, United Nations Human Development Report 2010.* New York: UNDP.

UNESCO (2009). *International Technical Guidance on Sexuality Education: An Evidence-informed Approach for Schools, Teachers and Health Educators.* Paris: UNESCO.

UNESCO and EDC. (2010). *Positive Partnerships: a Toolkit for the Greater Involvement of People Living with or Affected by HIV and AIDS in the Caribbean Education Sector.* Kingston, Jamaica: UNESCO and Newton, MA: EDC.

UNESCO and EDC (2005). *Leading the Way in the Education Sector: Advocating for a Comprehensive Approach to hiv and aids in the Caribbean.* Kingston, Jamaica: UNESCO and Newton MA: EDC.

UNICEF (2009). *Strengthening Health and Family Life Education in the Region: The Implementation, Monitoring and Evaluation of HFLE in Four CARICOM Countries.* Barbados: UNICEF.

UNICEF and UNFPA (2002). *Meeting Adolescent Development and Participation Rights: The Findings of Five Research Studies on Adolescents in Jamaica.* Kingston, Jamaica: UNICEF and UNFPA.

Walrond, E., and T. Roach (2006). "Barbados." In E. Beck et al. (eds), *The HIV Pandemic: Local and Global Implications.* Oxford: Oxford University Press.

Whitman, C. and Oomen, M. (2010). "Preliminary assessment of education ministries' capacity to address HIV and AIDS." In M. Morrissey, M. Bernard, and D. Bundy (eds), *Challenging HIV and AIDS: A New Role for Caribbean Education*. Kingston, Jamaica: *UNESCO*.

World Bank (2003). *Caribbean Youth Development: Issues and Policy Directions*. Washington, DC: World Bank .

— (2008). *Strengthening the Education Sector Response to HIV and AIDS in the Caribbean*. Washington, DC: World Bank.

HIV and the Internet Use: Sharing and Receiving Treatment Information

6

Fadhila Mazanderani and Jane Anderson

Chapter Outline

Introduction

In this chapter we analyze internet use as a form of HIV treatment education in the United Kingdom since the introduction of the highly active antiretroviral treatment (HAART). We draw on empirical research on how HIV positive women originally from sub-Saharan Africa, but currently living in the United Kingdom, use the internet to seek out and share treatment information. Instead of analyzing internet use in isolation, it is examined as embedded within the changing landscape of HIV treatment and care in the United Kingdom. Attention is drawn to how the provision of HIV treatment information has shifted in parallel with the changing availability and efficacy of HIV treatment. Within this we focus on how the various processes and sources of HIV treatment education do not operate in isolation, but mutually constitute each other. Moreover, it is argued that as the internet becomes an increasingly important source of health information, it too needs to be factored into how we understand both formal and informal learning processes in HIV care. Finally, we show how people living with HIV are not only the recipients of treatment information, but act in various different ways as critically important HIV treatment educators themselves, both online and offline.

The internet is an increasingly popular source of health information. Every day millions of people go online for health-related reasons: they seek out information; they rate health-care practitioners and hospitals; and they read about other people's experiences and share their own. Research consistently shows they feel this use has made a positive difference to their health. Yet, the rapid rise of the internet as a source for health information has not been met with universal approval.

While there has been considerable interest and promotion of the internet as a medium for patient empowerment, concern has been expressed as to whether, in practice, this use actually benefits people's health. The accuracy and completeness of online information has been questioned and, as more people and services go online, there is anxiety that instead of providing more equitable access to health services, differentials in internet access will become another form of health-care inequality. However, as research in the area of e-health has matured, it has become evident that the relationship between internet use and health outcomes is far from simple.

Statistically, internet use is associated with youth, higher levels of education, and higher incomes. Chronic illness, on the other hand, is linked to factors usually negatively correlated with internet use: being older, less educated, and having a lower socioeconomic status. Yet, once online, people living with chronic illness are particularly prolific e-health users. Surveys that measure the likelihood of someone using the internet in relation to health suggest that being female, not in full-time employment, engaged in other internet activities, working as a caregiver, and having specific medical concerns all increase the likelihood of its use for this purpose. On a more granular level, differences in use have been noted in relation to age, education, income, culture, ethnicity, ownership of private health insurance, and the presence of more than one health condition. This highlights how health-related internet use is contingent on and embedded in people's broader life worlds and environments of care. Building on this, in this chapter we examine the relationship between internet use, HIV care, and treatment education through the example of a specific group of women living with HIV in London.

Drawing on research on how 40 HIV-positive women, originally from 13 different sub-Saharan African countries but currently living in London, use the internet in relation to their health, we explore internet use as an alternative medium for learning about HIV treatment. Within this framework, we focus on the use of the internet to seek out different forms of treatment information and analyze how, instead of operating in isolation, these forms interact with and mutually constitute each other. A second key point we draw attention to through this case is the way in which people living with HIV are not only the recipients of knowledge, but play an active role, both formally and informally, in helping others learn about HIV. Thirdly, we show how, when analyzed from a broader perspective, learning about HIV has a salience that extends beyond more narrowly defined notions of patient choice and decision making and can, in their own way, be seen as form of "healing" for people living with the virus.

Before going into the main discussion, the work presented here is contextualized by a brief overview of existing research on internet use by people living with HIV. Next, we outline the methods used, followed by more background to the case study. The remainder of the chapter is structured as follows. First, internet use is embedded in the history of HIV treatment and information provision in the United Kingdom. Then, we look in some detail at the relationship between this use and other sources of HIV information. Finally, we analyze how women living with HIV spoke of the meaning that receiving and sharing treatment information had for them.

Researching internet use in the context of HIV/AIDS

Although the majority of adults and children diagnosed with HIV worldwide live in sub-Saharan Africa, the bulk of the research on internet use by people living with HIV has been carried out in "developed" countries, primarily North America and Western Europe. Given that the majority of people living in sub-Saharan Africa do not have access to the internet, this is perhaps not surprising, but it is also a reflection of a more general bias within e-health research to focus on "high-end" users—people who use the internet extensively and have home access. However, this trend has been changing and there has been an increased call for work that looks into how people with different levels of access use the internet in relation to their health. Indeed, this is essential if we are to try and understand how the people who most need better access to health-care services do or do not use information technology to achieve this.

Although the women who took part in this research were self-selected, based on their use of the internet for health-related purposes, they came from a range of educational and socioeconomic backgrounds, while their levels of internet familiarity and use differed greatly. This variety was intentional as we wanted to get a range of perspectives on internet use from those who used the internet every day to those who hardly used it at all. What we found was that not having internet access at home did not exclude women from using the internet and participants accessed the internet at a variety of different sites: community support groups, the library, internet cafés, and family and friend's houses. What emerged in relation to this was an appreciation for how where people used the internet shaped how they used it. Therefore, it is important to situate the question of internet use and its relationship to treatment education not only in terms of what was found online, but also in relation to the local specificities of its use. However, before going into the details of our study, in this section we contextualize it by looking briefly at other research on the use of the internet by people living with HIV.

Research on how people living with chronic illness use the internet has been carried out from a range of disciplinary perspectives: media and communications, sociology, education, health promotion, public health, health informatics, and psychology. The same can be said for research on how people living with HIV use the internet. This latter research has highlighted how the internet is used for a range of purposes that extend beyond what might be more narrowly defined as health related. An early piece of qualitative research on the use of the internet by people living with HIV found they used it for a variety of reasons: finding information, making social connections, as a form of advocacy, and as a means of escape (Reeves, 2001). In a later study, based on an analysis of websites created by people living with HIV, the internet was explored as a space of self-representation where four organizing themes emerged: autobiography, expertise, self-promotion, and dissent (Gillett, 2003). Work that focused more explicitly on the relationship between internet use and health outcomes for people living with HIV shed a positive light on the empowering potential of online health information and coping with illness (Kalichmen et al., 2003). However, this was subsequently modified with the caveat that patients do not always evaluate online information critically and may be vulnerable to misinformation online (Benotosch et al., 2004). Given the legacy of controversy surrounding HIV/AIDS activism, this is perhaps to be expected, and the use of the internet to propagate alternative or dissenting views has been a cause of some concern. Despite this, e-health research has shown how the websites with the strongest online presence usually belong to large incumbent health-care providers, nongovernment organizations, pharmaceutical companies, and insurers—a phenomenon referred to as "media convergence" (Seale, 2005). Moreover, work that has looked in more detail at how people living with chronic illness actually search for information online shows that they employ a range of verification practices and rarely trust what they find without corroborating it with other sources.

More generally, it has been suggested that the internet, in enabling people to educate themselves on information services with relative anonymity, has the potential to be a particularly privileged source of information on stigmatized illness.

The studies that have been carried out in relation to internet use by people living with HIV have adopted a range of methods. Like many studies on health and the media, a popular method has been to analyze the representation of people living with HIV online. This includes self-presentation in the form of blogs and forums, as well as how people living with HIV and the epidemic more generally are framed. People living with HIV have also been surveyed in relation to their internet use and, to a lesser extent, qualitative interviews have been carried out to try and understand in more detail the meaning that this use has for them in their lives. Very little work, however, has been done on how HIV-related websites and their content are produced.

Methods

This case study is based on research that explores how women, originally from sub-Saharan Africa, living with HIV in the United Kingdom, used the internet in relation to HIV and their health. It was important to contextualize the idea of internet use within the environment of HIV care and the variety of different information sources available. Of particular interest in this approach was the unpacking of the affective dimensions of this use. To explore these relationships, we conducted qualitative interviews with 40 women living with HIV. A major theme that emerged was that the women frequently searched online for HIV treatment information, by which we mean information pertaining specifically to highly active antiretroviral treatment (HAART) and associated medication.

Participants were recruited through three public HIV specialist outpatient centers in east London. 40 women from 13 sub-Saharan African countries (Angola, Burundi, Gambia, Ghana, Kenya, Nigeria, Sierra Leone, Somalia, South Africa, Uganda, Zambia, and Zimbabwe), receiving care at public-sector HIV specialist centers in east London, were recruited and interviewed about their information practices and internet use. The interviews were semi-structured: the first part was mostly unstructured, with participants talking retrospectively about their experiences of looking for health information and help, online and off-line, from the point they were diagnosed to the present. In the second half, specific questions were asked about the participant's history of and current use of the internet, and about how this use related to other sources of information.

Interviews were analyzed thematically in relation to internet use, HIV and health, and around those topics that emerged as particularly prominent in the interviews themselves. In addition to this thematic analysis, a strong emphasis was placed on analyzing how participants spoke of their use of the internet and its relationship to other sources of information.

In addition, two focus groups were carried out, within community support groups, with people living with HIV who had not participated in a one-on-one interview. The main themes from the research interviews were used as prompts. The aim of this was to extend the findings, but also to test their validity. Online information providers and representatives from community groups were also interviewed, both formally and informally, and these interviews and associated field notes were analyzed in conjunction with the patient interviews. A document analysis was performed on information provided in hard copy to patients in clinics as well as online. The online information analyzed was based on the websites mentioned by interview participants as well as Google searches carried out on 100 popular HIV-related search terms. Based on the websites returned by these searches, a web-link analysis was performed using the Issue Crawler software made available by govcom.org.

Context and case

While HIV infections acquired in the United Kingdom are still mostly among men who have sex with men (MSM), there are reports of increasing numbers of diagnoses among ethnic minorities, women, and relatively recent immigrants. Diagnoses among these groups have broadly mirrored the worldwide prevalence of HIV, in which the majority of those being diagnosed come from Africa, and sub-Saharan Africa, in particular. Moreover, over half of those diagnosed in 2008 had a CD4 count below 350 within three months of their diagnosis. This means, according to UK clinical recommendations, that treatment should start immediately.

Research on the African community of the United Kingdom and HIV/ AIDS shows three recurring themes (Prost et al., 2008). First, African patients frequently receive their HIV positive diagnosis at an advanced stage of disease progression and, as a result, are often very unwell at the time and have associated co-infections such as tuberculosis (TB). Secondly, in addition to their medical concerns, these patients often face difficulties with immigration status, social isolation, discrimination and stigma, all of which act as barriers to accessing health care and social services. Thirdly, they experience high levels of unemployment and poverty, which compound these issues. All three of these themes were reiterated by the women who took part in this research, in which they spoke of being diagnosed with HIV as just one struggle among many daily issues.

As the demographics of people diagnosed with HIV in the United Kingdom shifted, the health-care services had to adjust as well. A greater investment of resources originally created to tailor education, testing, and treatment of African immigrants, largely by the United Kingdom's Department of Health but other organizations as well, now included the creation of new organizations, such as the African HIV Policy Network (AHPN) (Weatherburn et al., 2003). It was recognized that health-care practitioners had to deal with radically new issues, such as extreme cultural and linguistic diversity, and the social issues their patients faced, such as extreme poverty and histories of trauma and sociopolitical upheaval.

For the women who took part in this research, their experience of living with HIV in the United Kingdom sits at the intersection of an "African" and a "British" one, resulting in highly variable interpretations of what it means to be a person living with HIV (Flowers et al., 2006). On the one hand, they receive free treatment and care in a country where, because of access to HAART, HIV is no longer a death sentence, but a chronic illness. At the same time, many of them still associate HIV with the context of their home countries where HIV is a frequent cause of death, and in many cases they have lost family members, including husbands and children. Moreover, some of these women were unsure how long they could remain in the United Kingdom because of their unstable immigration status, and the lack of treatment in their home countries was a real issue.

The participants of this study were primarily well educated and placed a high importance on having access to information and knowledge, paralleling similar studies on this topic (Doyal and Anderson, 2005). In addition to the importance placed on acquiring information *for* better health, participants also stressed the importance of their day-to-day management of information *about* their health as a mechanism for managing stigma. For example, they would report the importance of managing information about their HIV positive diagnosis in order to prevent those in their home countries from knowing about it.

All the women who participated in this study were receiving care at a public-sector, specialist, HIV outpatient center. In the United Kingdom the majority of HIV treatment and care is carried out at such centers. This meant that they were provided with education about their disease by specialist HIV physicians and nurses during appointments and they had access to information in the form of magazines and information leaflets in the clinic. Additionally, they had access to a number of community groups operating in the United Kingdom, which provide support services for people living with HIV including help with immigration and employment issues as well as emotional support and counseling. For these women, therefore, the internet was one of many sources of information on HIV/AIDS treatment. Understanding this broader context is important for understanding *how*, *when*, and *what* information women searched for online, as well as *what they found*.

The changing dynamics of HIV treatment and information in the United Kingdom

Since the introduction of HAART in 1996 there has been a major reduction in HIV-related morbidity and mortality in the United Kingdom. The emergence of treatment for HIV, but not a cure, has meant that the provision of information around the virus has focused increasingly on managing the disease and managing the delivery of therapy (Rosengarten et al., 2004). Initially, treatment regimes were extremely complex and required patients to take multiple drugs throughout the day. While this has improved, living with HIV in the era of HAART has given rise to new challenges centered on balancing treatment benefits and risks, such as distressing side effects including diarrhea, nausea and vomiting, skin rashes, and sexual problems, as well as serious implications for patients' health, such as peripheral neuropathy, liver and kidney toxicity, lipodystrophy, and lipoatrophy. As these drugs, and the treatment around them, shape HIV as a chronic condition, new questions are arising: How should we deal with HIV treatment in an aging population? How should safe conception and prevention of mother-to-child transmission be best managed? What are the consequences of a lifetime of medication for the first generation of young adults born HIV positive? What are the questions about HIV treatment we need to ask beyond those of access to medication and compliance with treatment regimes? These were some of the questions that women living with HIV are going online to ask.

For example, a woman who was over 50 years old and who had been on ART for more than ten years wanted to find out about the consequences of medication on the lives of older women. Another woman, who was currently undergoing fertility treatment, searched the internet in order to know more about her chances for success in giving birth to an HIV-negative child. A pregnant mother, before agreeing to take medication to help prevent mother-to-child transmission, went on Youtube.com to look for videos of children whose mothers had taken the same medication that was being prescribed for her to ensure they were developing normally. A young woman who had been born HIV positive and had been on medication for 12 years wanted to find out more about research to find a cure and, in doing so, discover whether she had the possibility of a "normal" future before deciding if there was any point in enrolling at a university. These are just some examples that illustrate how what participants searched for online was shaped by the changing nature of HIV treatment available in the United Kingdom. Significantly, what they *found* was similarly shaped by the way in which the provision of HIV-treatment information has evolved in the United Kingdom.

While HIV/AIDS is not the first health condition to have received large-scale media attention, the media have played a very prominent and often-criticized role in its history. During the early years of the epidemic, there was, and still is, a great deal of misinformation, stigma, and prejudice dissemination through various media channels. In response, one of the key aims of the AIDS organizations that emerged during this early period was to provide appropriate information and support to those affected. However, as the epidemic has changed, so too have the types of information and services provided in relation to it and many of these organizations are now online.

From their very inception, HIV organizations in the United Kingdom, such as the Terrence Higgins Trust (THT), actively leveraged different media forms to provide HIV-related information. By the end of 1983, THT was distributing its first educational and prevention leaflets on AIDS, an activity that continues across a range of mediums: leaflets, magazines, phone support, face-to-face support and, as of 1996, the internet. Similarly, the National AIDS Manual (NAM), which was set up in 1987 to provide HIV/AIDS-related information and support, has been online since 1998. The provision of HIV/AIDS information, to the public at large and to those more directly affected, continues to be a core activity of HIV/AIDS organizations, and there are a number of organizations based in the United Kingdom, such as NAM and i-Base, the explicit purpose of which is to provide treatment information to people living with HIV. Indeed, when compared to other serious health conditions, there is considerably more information about HIV online, a great deal of which is rated by HIV clinicians as being of excellent quality (Krakower et al., 2010). What this means is that a lot of HIV treatment information on the internet is being collected and organized by technically savvy people, many of whom are living with HIV.

In addition to the way in which internet use is embedded in the changing nature of HIV treatment and the historical contingency of HIV information provision in the United Kingdom, the internet comprises multiple different information sources and technologies. Moreover, the internet was only one multidimensional information resource among many. Even among avid internet users, research participants spoke of how they sought out treatment information from a range of different sources, contrasting and collating the information they found. While HIV physicians were usually the preferred source of treatment information, participants read information booklets, phoned HIV community organizations' help-lines, and spoke to other people living with HIV through a variety of media. Rather than the internet being used to replace face-to-face consultations with doctors, it was primarily seen as a means *to enhance* the information received in consultations.

The women we interviewed also frequently prepared for consultations by looking for information online. For example, one participant searched for the symptoms she was experiencing in order to have an idea of what the possible treatments would be before making her appointment with her doctor. Another used it after her consultation to find further information on possible side effects of the drug that had been prescribed for her. Significantly, however, participants rarely spoke of using the internet to *challenge* their HIV physicians or other sources of more official "medical" knowledge. Yet, this did not mean that these various sources of information were interchangeable. Even when participants said they found the *same information*, the form the information came in had implications for the meaning it took on for them. In the section that follows we look in a little more detail at how research participants spoke of different ways of knowing about HIV in relation to different sources and processes of HIV treatment education.

The internet as a "new" source of HIV treatment information to support education

As with any "new" technology, there has been a considerable interest in how use of the internet for health will change patient-doctor relations and the general meaning of patienthood. However, as argued in the previous section, the internet is very much embedded within existing sources of health information and health-care environments. In this section we look at the question of what is new about the use of the internet for HIV treatment education. In order to think through some potential aspects of the novelty of e-health and HIV education, we turn first to the question of how internet use interacts with existing patient-doctor relations.

HIV physicians were perceived by most participants as being their primary source of HIV treatment information. Yet this was not the case for other medical specializations. Indeed, strong feelings were expressed with regards to other practitioners and areas of medicine, especially general practitioners:

> You know, doctors who are dealing with HIV, they are okay, but GPs they need an education. I have been insulted left, right and centre by my own GP. (Interview participant)

In some cases participants felt they were well provided for with regards to HIV treatment information, but found it more problematic to get support in relation to general health queries.

The distinctions participants drew between different areas of medicine are salient for our analysis here because they highlight the variable nature of HIV/AIDS education, even within the field of medicine. Rather, how people searched for information and what they then did with that information was situated within relationships with specific medical experts, such as their HIV physician, but also in relation to domains of health care and their associated practices. This is important because, as the disease burden of countries such as the United Kingdom shift from acute to chronic conditions, there is a strong interest in finding cost-effective ways of supporting people living with these conditions. One way this has manifested itself is in the emphasis placed on patient decision making and responsibility in health care. However, how patients go about becoming informed, why they do so, and if they can, indeed, make a decision based on the information they find, cannot be separated out from the health-care practices in which they are situated. Assuming the field of clinical medicine is uniform and that patients engage with medical information in an abstract or generic way simplifies this process by brushing over crucial complexities that impinge on patients' health care and associated information practices. Being informed is not simply about what you know; how you know, and in relation to whom, is often just as important. The same holds for the relationship between internet use and health education.

The internet is not one technology. It is a collection of different websites, services and information, and although we have been referring it to as one unit, it is in fact made up of many information technologies. This plurality is reflected in the way in which different websites and services were used in relation to HIV/AIDS. Sometimes participants went directly to the websites of major HIV treatment information providers, the URLs for which were often provided on information booklets in the clinic. Sometimes they went to HIV forums, read, and posted questions. Information found on blogs was not considered the same as that found on pharmaceutical websites. Among these different uses, however, one technology emerged as particularly important: search engines.

All the women who took part in this study relied heavily on Google.com to search for information online. Indeed, for many of them Google was the internet. When asked how they used the internet the answer was frequently just, "Google." The salience for understanding what has been referred to as "the political economy of search engines" has been raised in relation to a number of different areas of internet use and is highly relevant with regards to HIV information. Search engines need to be included not simply as a tool for finding information, but as an active participant in online treatment education. Our interviews show that not only the reliance on Google for searches, but that the results of those searches, or specifically their order, was important in what information was accessed. Participants frequently used the same, well-established sources, from different search engines, because these web pages were listed in the first page of results:

> When I go to the internet for some reason I trust the information. I do. Uhm [pause] because they are different, even if you Google, it will come up with different websites and then you read through the first one and then you read through the second one and you try and connect the information and it adds up. So, simple examples like, if you enter 'urinary tract infection,' which I did in the past, you get the same, almost the same information, signs and symptoms. You go on another one and you get the same information. It's not confusing . . . (Interview participant)

However, even if in some cases, such as the example above, this information was perceived as "almost the same," and although the content is important, the practices that went into the internet search are the main point of interest here. By facilitating the activities of search and comparison, search engines such as Google have emerged as playing a vital role in how people learn about HIV treatment information. Our study shows that while the information itself is not new, the relationships between different sources of knowledge and ways of knowing shift and reassemble, depending on how search engines are used.

Different sources of information were approached and assimilated by participants in different ways and through different media. Not only did participants' use of different technologies shape what they found, but their desire for treatment education changed over time. Instead of the internet replacing other forms of treatment education, part of its importance came about in terms of how it related to other sources of information.

> Because it's my health. It's me that understands myself better than the doctor and I have to take charge of my own health. All the doctor does is to ask how are you feeling? He gives me treatment, I go home [pause]. But all the other things that I need to know? That I need to check for myself, the doctor cannot do that one. He is not paid to do all that. So he will just do his own bit, so this one is my own bit. I have to check for it. Because it's good that we have internet, it's good that we have a lot of information on the internet, and maybe some of it is not good, but at least it will give you a rough idea and once you have a rough idea you take the matter up to someone who knows. (Interview participant)

In the next section, we move from talking about patients as those seeking HIV treatment information to looking at how they were also often the providers of this information.

Sharing and receiving HIV treatment information

As is well known, people living with HIV do not simply receive treatment information; they are actively engaged in producing and disseminating it. Indeed, HIV/AIDS has become the archetype condition cited in relation to patient activism. One result of this ongoing legacy of HIV patient activism is that a great deal of the information produced and distributed to patients in clinical settings has been collected and packaged by people living with HIV. Moreover, people living with HIV frequently volunteer and work in community organizations, educating others about HIV. This is very much in evidence on the internet, where people living with HIV keep blogs, participate in forums, exchange stories about their experiences and work in more formal capacities on treatment information websites. They are active in numerous ways, ranging from high profile advocacy to other, less visible, but nonetheless highly important, activities.

For many of the women who took part in this research, practices of educating other people about HIV were an important aspect of their internet use. In some cases this meant the internet was used in order to find out more on a certain topic that was then subsequently shared with others. This often happened when internet users at community groups met others who were less able, due to language barriers or other difficulties, to find and understand HIV treatment information. However, finding information developed by others and disseminating it more widely was only one aspect of these sharing practices. In addition to this, participants were particularly keen to share their own experiences of treatment. This type of experiential knowledge was highly privileged and was seen as something that only other people living with HIV could provide ". . . because they have suffered it. They are now talking from experience, so they will tell you, 'This drug, don't even attempt it, even if your doctor suggests this one, just refuse.' It's not good." Central as learning about treatment was to these acts of educating each other, it was also a means of creating a sense of community and belonging. In some cases this resulted in life-changing decisions. One participant decided to embark on a social-work degree after meeting other women living with HIV who were engaged in higher education. Another decided she would try and get pregnant after reading about how HIV-positive women had successfully given birth to HIV-negative children. A third decided to stay in the United Kingdom as she had been so inspired by the positive and welcoming attitudes of the women she had met in a community group. This experiential information was used in conjunction with information received from different sources, such as side-effects information provided with the drugs:

> I read about other people's experiences and it is quite good. I even go to the library to read about it. When I get new medication I go and look because if you read the leaflet with the side effects and you take a book where research has been done in some part of the world and people are talking about their experiences and their side effects, then you realize I am not the only one having this problem. (Interview participant)

While this information had practical implications (in terms of decision making about treatment and managing side effects), it clearly also had very strong affective ones. In some instances, even when information had been provided by health-care practitioners, hearing other people's stories brought about a sense of reassurance. Being able to talk about these experiences was described by one participant as the point at which she started to accept her diagnosis and "to begin to heal". Just as using search engines allowed for new forms of comparison through practices of search and retrieval, sharing stories allowed our research participants to compare themselves to others living with HIV: "It gives me courage and I learn more that sometimes I don't know that I have to do this and do that and I can cope or this one was like me. I was like this. I compare myself to some people." Use of the internet was particularly significant in relation to the sharing of experiences for women who were unable to attend community groups. In many cases this was due to their fear of other people finding out about their HIV positive status, or because family members or partners did not want them to attend these groups. These women often used the internet in order to help other people dealing with an HIV-positive diagnosis:

> because sometimes your story can help someone who has been wanting to go for a test for a long time and they, they're scared.
> I want to preach something which I know I am going through and which I can understand when someone is in my face and they are telling me what they are going through. I think with that knowledge I can help someone.(Interview participant)

Conclusions

While studies of "new" technologies often fall prey to utopian or dystopian images of how it might or might not bring about a certain future, in reality the situation is far more complex. By basing this chapter on empirical research on the use of internet technologies among a specific group of women, our aim is not to generalize these local findings, but rather to explore some of the local specificities of that use.

In this chapter we focused on the use of the internet as a form of HIV treatment education. Rather than looking at the internet as something "new," it was analyzed as embedded in the changing context of HIV treatment and care in the United Kingdom. Of particular interest was how the salience of internet use emerged in relation to, rather than as a replacement of, other sources of treatment information. Moreover, we argued that when talking about process of learning about HIV treatment, it is important to not only look at it narrowly as facilitating practical decision making, but also to include an appreciation for its many affective dimensions. Some of the dimensions highlighted here were how the sharing of experiential information built up communities and strong bonds between women living with HIV, often inspiring a sense of hope and acceptance.

As more and more people gain access to HAART it becomes increasingly necessary to understand the different ways in which people use information and educational processes in relation to living with HIV. Similarly, as internet access expands and service providers, for a variety of reasons, provide more information and services online, it is necessary to understand the use of the internet in people's everyday lives and health-care practices. Nowhere is this more pertinent than in relation to the shifting parameters of HIV as a chronic illness and the management of complex pharmacological regimes.

Questions for reflection

1. How does the changing nature of "education" in light of new technologies impact how we think about HIV/AIDS education?
2. What are the different ways these women used the internet to acquire information? How does the use of different search engines impact this educational act?
3. How might new information technologies impact HIV/AIDS education in the context and region of your focus?

Reference list

Benotsch, E., S. Kalichman, and L. Weinhardt (2004). "HIV-AIDS patients' evaluation of health information on the internet: the digital divide and vulnerability to fraudulent claims." *Journal of Consulting and Clinical Psychology* 72 (6): 1004–11.

Doyal, L., and J. Anderson (2005). "'My fear is to fall in love again': how HIV-positive African women survive in London." *Social Science and Medicine* 60: 1729–38.

Flowers, P.., M. Davis, G. Hart, M. Rosengarten, J. Frankis and J. Imrie (2006). "Diagnosis and stigma and identity amongst HIV-positive black Africans living in the UK." *Psychology and Health* 21 (1): 109–22.

Gillett, J. (2003). "Media activism and internet use by people with HIV/AIDS." *Sociology of Health and Illness* 25 (6): 608–24.

Kalichman, S., E. Benotsch, L. Weinhardt, J. Austin, L. Webster, and C. Chauncey (2003). "Health-related internet use, coping, social support, and health indicators in people living with hiv/aids: preliminary results from a community survey." *Health Psychology* 22 (1): 111–16.

Krakower, D., C. K. Kwan, D. S. Yassa, and R. A. Colvin (2010). "Surfing the web: iAIDS: HIV-related internet resources for the practicing clinician." *Clinical Infectious Diseases* 51 (7): 813–22.

Prost, A., J. Elford, J. Imrie, M. Petticrew and G. Hart (2008). "Social, behavioural, and intervention research among people of sub-Saharan African origin living with HIV in the UK and Europe: literature review and recommendations for intervention." *AIDS Behaviour* 12: 170–94.

Reeves, P. (2001). "How individuals coping with HIV/AIDS use the internet." *Health Education Research* 16 (6): 709–19.

Rosengarten, M, J. Imrie, P. Flowers, M. Davis and G. Hart(2004). "After the euphoria: HIV medical technologies from the perspective of their prescribers." *Sociology of Health and Illness* 26 (5): 575–96.

Seale, C. (2005). "New directions for critical internet health studies: representing cancer experience on the web." *Sociology of Health and Illness* 27(4): 515–40.

Weatherburn, P., W. Ssanyu-Seruma, and F. Hickson (2003). *Project NASAH: An Investigation into the HIV Treatment, Information and Other Needs of African People with HIV Resident in England.* London: Sigma Research.

HIV/AIDS Education in Turkey

7

Tuncay Ergene and Kerim Munir

Chapter Outline

Introduction

Nearly half of the population of Turkey is under 25 years with the median age range of 15 to 49 considered as the most at-risk group for HIV infection. The population's knowledge of sexually transmitted infections (STIs), as a facilitating factor for HIV transmission, remains limited, and a major public health challenge. The most common type of transmission in Turkey is among HIV discordant heterosexual, homosexual, and bisexual pairs, as well as intravenous drug users. The disease is not epidemic among the general population. Condom use among sexually active youth is low. However, since Turkey is predominantly Muslim, male circumcision is almost universal and helps in reducing transmission. The rapid expansion of tourism in recent years has led to an increase in the number of visitors from countries that have high rates of HIV/AIDS (UNAIDS, 2003). In addition, a large number of young Turkish people working abroad are at high risk of becoming infected and bringing HIV home. By the end of 2009, Turkey had a cumulative total of 2,315 reported AIDS cases with just over half from heterosexual partners, around 8 percent from homosexual partners and around 2 percent in children and adolescents 15 years of age or under. About 7 percent of those infected with HIV caught the virus from sharing needles, with the rise in these infections mirroring the rise in intravenous drug use in Turkey in recent years.

The national education sector in Turkey has a strong potential to make a difference in the fight against HIV/AIDS. It offers an organized and efficient way to reach large numbers of school-age youth representing groups either most at risk (secondary education) or most receptive to efforts that seek to influence behavior (primary education). Furthermore, secondary, and higher (tertiary) education provides an effective means to reach a portion of the population that is important not in terms of numbers, but as a crucial resource of productive human capital for a country. As such, it affords a critical opportunity to scale up successful approaches, vital in view of the wide and rapid reach of the epidemic. In addition, the sector's reach extends to two other important groups: teachers and communities (including parents) who can play a crucial role in efforts to address the problem at its roots.

A well-publicized national case of a boy infected with HIV has led to media attention on Turkey's HIV/AIDS epidemic, otherwise a rare focus of national interest since the incidence of HIV infections is perceived to be relatively low. The child in question was infected as a newborn. As his HIV status became known he was then denied access to education at his local primary school. The father of the boy reacted by noting that as a citizen of the republic his child ought to benefit from what he considered to be his child's natural right to education under the constitution. Such a universal response could have come from a parent anywhere in the world whose child is unfairly denied access to schooling because of a stigmatizing condition. In this case the condition in question was HIV. Many developing countries like Turkey, especially those that are predominantly Muslim and undergoing social and economic changes, face unique social challenges in relation to HIV/AIDS. Restriction of educational opportunities is a part of such an adverse response. This chapter will explore the contextual reasons wherein education is important both directly and indirectly in not only decreasing the impact of existing HIV infections in the country but also in preventing future infections. In this chapter we argue that in openly discussing stigma attached to HIV/AIDS, peer education efforts remain as one of the most promising interventions, particularly among youth facing challenges in accepting differences in their experience of sexuality (Ergene et al., 2005). We further argue that HIV status impacts not only inclusive education rights but human rights. Inclusive education is therefore a full-fledged part of a humanitarian response to adversity including infections, disasters, and social adversity. The debate has wider social policy implications as it takes into account political, cultural, and economic conditions in the country.

Despite great progress in the expansion of compulsory education in the country, even without HIV/AIDS, the education sector faces major challenges in Turkey; more than 800,000 children aged 6 to 12 are out of school, two-thirds of them, girls. The tremendous potential of education and the crippling impact on societies of the HIV/AIDS epidemic presents an enormous opportunity to act and a grave danger if they do not. This divergent path is most evident in Turkey where the predominance of youth in the population promises particularly rich rewards for an education-focused strategy, but dire consequences if a passive strategy succumbs to the vicious cycle engendered by HIV/AIDS (Kontas, 2003).

In this chapter, we also present a developmental perspective to HIV/AIDS. We highlight the work with students in prevention of HIV/AIDS, especially in the context of developmentally informed psychoeducational programs. We discuss the educational, legal, and ethical aspects of HIV/AIDS: role of teachers and school administrators, the positive impact of parental involvement, and prevention of stigma related to HIV/AIDS in school settings.

Conditions in Turkey

Turkey is strategically situated at the crossroads of Europe and Asia. The country shares land borders with eight countries; the Mediterranean Sea and the island of Cyprus are located to the south. This geographical context has historically made Turkey a natural pathway for immigrants and increasing tourism. Both these factors are also known to increase HIV infections. In addition to this, increasing numbers of citizens working abroad regularly return home, sometimes bringing the virus with them. Other contributory factors that increase the risk of STIs include: the irregular medical examinations of women working in brothels; the high number of unregistered sexual workers; and the scarcity of condom use in sexual relationships. In 2004, when the estimated population of Turkey was 65 million citizens, the ministry of health reported the number of HIV-infected individuals in Turkey to be 3,989. However, the true prevalence of HIV infections in the general population is not known due to the lack of an adequate HIV surveillance system. This lack of data also makes it difficult to determine the real status of STIs and to take the requisite preventive measures in Turkey (Ay and Karabey, 2006). Because most HIV transmissions occur between people engaging in heterosexual relationships, with increasing numbers sharing needles, it is important to prevent the spread among the general population with educational programs playing a paramount role to reach a wide range of young people, as well as high-risk groups.

Although 97 percent of the population is Muslim, secular laws provide an open and free environment for relationships, particularly in the light of the very rapid rural-to-urban migration in recent years. Even so, a variety of sexual attitudes and behaviors still exist, based on different sociocultural groups, ethnicity, gender and urban rural distinctions, age groupings, and educational level. In rural areas, where 35 percent of the Turkish people currently live, traditional conservative values still prevail. There has also been an influx of conservative sexual attitudes and behaviors because of increased migration from rural to urban centers. Discussing sex is still largely a taboo for the majority of Turks, irrespective of urban or rural residence, and premarital sex often is not socially permissible for women. These prohibitions may sometimes result in involuntary hymen examinations, compulsory marriages of young people after premarital sex, or violence against and sometimes murder of women who break with tradition (Çelikbaş et al., 2008; Duyan and Yildirim, 2003). For men, in contrast, a more open sexuality is permitted including extramarital affairs. Such a social milieu highlights gender roles in sexual behavior and attitudes (Ayrancı, 2005).

Education

The cultural taboo of talking about sexuality is reflected in the general lack of sex education in schools. Most established curricula do not include sufficient information, either for teachers or for students, on sexual and reproductive issues. In some developed countries, sexual education, adjusted to the age and needs of the child, is provided from the first years of primary school. In Turkey its content is analogous to instruction on "the reproductive system of plants" in primary school and "the reproductive system of males and females" in high school. One of the main impediments to sexual education is said to be the cultural reserve of educators and parents in these matters. This reserve shapes social attitudes with preference given to waiting until the child starts a discussion and asks questions. Many do not feel confident about answering possible questions, fear giving too much information too early, and worry about inadvertently suggesting sexual experimentation (Gökengin, 2002). In such an atmosphere many youngsters inevitably avoid any conversation about sexuality, either because it risks embarrassment, or they are simply unsure about how their elders may judge them. Nevertheless, research shows that older children, adolescents, and young adults want education about sexuality and reproductive issues as part of the school curriculum. As a result of this deficit, the main sources of information about sexual matters for children and adolescents remain their friends and the media, which paradoxically also remain the main sources of information for parents and teachers as well.

Compared to previous generations, there is evidence that the current youth are becoming increasingly sexually active (Cok et al., 2001). The social, cultural, and economic context that contemporary young Turks live in is a *perfect storm* where STIs encounter HIV. This rapid sociocultural change clashes with the lack of educational response, making the negative side effects seen in other similar contexts a serious risk. Those who study this context and possible educational responses argue for peer education as an appropriate intervention in Turkey (Aras et al., 2007; Eylen, 1996; Ozcebe et al., 2004; Ozeruz, 1999). University students in major cities are particularly at higher risk for HIV infection for a number of reasons: many become more sexually active as they move to urban settings, away from their families, and engage in sexual experimentation and unprotected sex. In a study of Turkish university students, the average age reported for their first sexual intercourse was 17, contrary to the widespread belief of most Turkish citizens that most youth wait to be married before engaging in sexual activity (Çok et al., 2001). In a sample of 530 undergraduates, 36.6 percent of male and 12.7 percent of female university students reported that they had premarital sex. Other studies show that university students in Turkey engage in more risky sexual behavior as a result of peer pressure, use of alcohol and drugs, feelings of embarrassment about sexuality, and lack of opportunities to meet sexual partners privately. Ergene et al. (2005) investigated the impact of both peer education and single-session educational lectures on subsequent HIV/AIDS knowledge, attitude, and practices (KAPs) among university students. Results showed that there was a statistically significant difference in student KAPs compared to the control group. Male and female students in both intervention groups showed improved attitudinal scores toward HIV/AIDS compared with students in the control group.

Peer education interventions are a strategy frequently utilized for preventing HIV infections and other sexually transmitted infections (STIs) worldwide (Backett-Milburn and Wilson, 2000). Such interventions select individuals who share demographic characteristics (e.g., by age and gender) or risk behaviors with a target group (e.g. commercial sex work, or intravenous drug use). The intervention starts by training these peer educators to increase awareness, impart knowledge, and encourage behavior change among members of that same group. Peer education can be delivered formally in structured settings, such as classrooms, but also informally as part of everyday interactions. Peer educators can have a strong influence on individual behavior because they have a much higher level of trust and comfort with the target groups, allowing for more open discussion on sensitive topics and greater efficacy in knowledge transfer (Campbell and MacPhail, 2002; Turhan et al., 2006;). Peer educators also have much better access to inaccessible populations that may have limited interaction with more traditional health programs because of stigma, fear, or sociocultural mores. For example, young and unmarried women are more likely to discuss reproductive health with other females of similar age without suspicion of premarital sex than publicly visit an STI clinic or prenatal clinic. Peer-education programs empower both the educator and the target group by creating a sense of solidarity and collective action (Campbell and Mzaidume, 2001; Milburn, 1995). Interventions using peers can also be more cost effective than interventions that rely on highly trained professional staff (Aggleton and Warwick, 2002).

There are a handful of studies that have utilized or evaluated peer-education interventions in Turkey (Babadogan, 2002; Ergene et al., 2005; Gökengin, 2002; Özcebe et al., 2004). Zeren (2005) employed "play acting" as a natural communication tool to reach students in her research. A recent meta-analysis of the effectiveness of peer education interventions for HIV prevention in developing countries (Medley et al., 2009) indicate that these programs are moderately effective at improving behavioral outcomes, but that there is no conclusive evidence of an increase in the number of people getting tested for HIV-related symptoms. In Turkey, most people who test positive for HIV infection are only incidentally identified by authorities: they are patients, hospitalized for another illness or vague symptoms, and during a bout of complicated illness are offered testing for a range of problems which happen to include HIV.

Landmark case of an HIV-infected boy

The effects of HIV infections among school-aged children captured the attention of the public a decade ago. Turkey is going through a rite of passage in dealing with the responsibility of caring for HIV-infected youngsters. This has in some ways been a difficult learning curve and is exemplified by the plight of a seven-year-old boy, mentioned earlier, who received an HIV-infected blood transfusion when he was 20 days old. As background, every year in Turkey there is a need for 1.5 million units of blood, with only 1.1 million units collected, thus leaving a national deficit of 0.4 million units. There are close to 300 blood donation centers in the country, but no common standard for screening has yet been instituted. Examples of individuals contracting viral infections including HIV therefore greatly contribute to public fears. Ornek Büken (2006) explained this loss of trust and cooperation in the experience of one family of an HIV-infected boy in emphasizing his right for an inclusive education. The youngster was born prematurely in a public city hospital in the western part of the country where he acquired the infection through a blood transfusion at a Turkish Red Crescent Blood Center. He was diagnosed with HIV infection some eight months later. By 1998, a legal case was brought by the family against Turkish Red Crescent and led to a large financial settlement for the family, which is highly unusual in Turkey (Radikal, 2010). When the child was ready to enter primary school in his neighborhood, other parents became aware of his status and objected to him attending the same school as their children, fearing that he might infect them. In response to this situation—initially the provincial education director, and subsequently the provincial governor's office—felt obliged to intervene. Staff from the ministry of education and the Guidance and Research Center (charged for providing psychosocial and special educational supports to students and families) met with the students and their families. The other parents requested that the child with HIV infection be educated separately or sent to a special school. The ministry of education's local authorities tried to address the demands.

The infected child's parents became increasingly upset and made their discontent clear to the authorities. They felt that that the authorities were not providing them adequate support to ensure their son's full participation in everyday school life. They were also angry at the other parents for ostracizing their son; they insisted that their goal was to secure their child's right to education. In so doing, they also requested support from physicians to make it known that the virus was not contagious in the school setting as long as proper precautions were implemented. They complained to the school principal and teachers that they were not adequately prepared to protect their son's rights. They felt the school authorities simply did not have any experience or specialized knowledge on HIV to handle the situation before it got out of control.

Although initially they insisted that their son attend the school, as they faced more resistance and stigma by other parents, they decided to hold their son back from the school fearing repercussions. They felt obliged to make up untrue stories and present excuses for keeping him away from school.

Subsequent developments led them to decide to take the case to court and to declare that their son had a right to education. If access was not to be provided, they declared that they would take the case to the European Commission on Human Rights. They refused the offer of home schooling or education in a health-care setting. They also indicated that the boy was having difficulty speaking and stuttering. One group of parents awaiting the court's ruling indicated that they were indeed very sorry for the family's situation but that they too had rights. They asked the boy's parents to consider what they would if they were in the other parents' situation. They expressed their fears about the risk of their children becoming HIV infected. They indicated that they too were simply trying to protect their children's rights (Milliyet, 2003).

The lawyer representing the boy argued that the boy had a right to education in a public-school setting, emphasizing that HIV was not infectious through ordinary means of contact, especially if adequate precautions had been taken. The court relied on a report by a commission at the faculty of medicine's hospital and the provincial health directorate, decreeing that the HIV virus was not contagious in the classroom. This ruling was followed by a statement from the ministry of education that the boy would continue his education in the normal manner with his peers. The parents, although happy about the court's decision, were still concerned about the reactions of the other parents and feared repercussions if he returned to the school.

The case became a landmark that brought HIV/AIDS to the forefront of public discourse with ethical, legal, and even political implications. The results show that in situations relating to public fear and stigma governments need to act decisively (Ornek Büken, 2006). The case was unique in Turkey in that the family was awarded a record-high financial compensation for the

Blood Transfusion Center error (Radikal, 2010). The issue of fear and stigma was probably the most prominent aspect of the case. The situation could not be resolved until legal supports intervened to protect the child's right to education. The legal precedent in this case also facilitated future government policy around treatment of not only school-aged children with HIV, but all individuals with HIV/AIDS in the country (Akyuz, 2000).

There continues to be limited attention given to HIV/AIDS prevention in the national education system in Turkey. Teachers and school administrators need to be updated with relevant information. Students need to receive education based on their developmental level and relevant preventive activities carried out in the schools with the full knowledge of the parents. In the case of HIV-positive students, administrators should provide support to the affected students and their parents. Teachers and school administrators should always keep in mind that they are role models within the school community. The school administration should sponsor service training sessions and seminars for teachers. School counselors should be trained in providing support for students and parents with outreach counseling and guidance services to the school community as may be necessary (Zeren and Ergene, 2008).

Gender disparities

In many other countries, as in Turkey, the attitudes toward an individuals' plight with HIV/AIDS are principally a question of human rights and respect for human dignity (Ornek Büken, 2006). As professionals in the education and mental health field, we also play a specific and important part in the the the need for definitive action. The ecological nature of human rights means that a threat to one person is a threat to all. The social stigma attached to HIV/AIDS, which still exists globally, as exemplified by this case, was magnified in Turkey because of the lack of education and common cultural and religious taboos relating to sexual behavior. Stigma surrounding even suspicion of permissive sexuality is intense; the affected individuals can be shunned by the entire family as well as by the community. This means that individuals engaging in risky sexual behaviors are forced into secrecy because of the fear of the stigma their actions could bring, and they are extremely unlikely to be forthcoming in seeking appropriate voluntary counseling, testing, and treatment. In the case of Turkey, extreme stigma creates barriers to successful implementation of prevention and treatment strategies even where they are available. These factors continue to lead to the significant underreporting of the rate of HIV infections in the country (Kontas, 2003). Turkey is a traditional society with an imbalance in power between men and women; this imbalance extends beyond sexual relationships in society. In most cases, men have greater power and voice than women, making private home life a sanctuary for many women. Women have less educational opportunity than their male counterparts. Although the male–female disparity is decreasing in many walks of life, there is less access to societal resources, and less attribution of civil, legal, and sexual rights. Due to these inequalities, women are particularly susceptible to contracting HIV/AIDS as they are less likely to be able to negotiate with infected partners. Women are also easy targets in abusive relationships and are less able to have access to treatment resources or cope with illness once infected.

Changing social landscapes and prevention of stigma

With a surge in economic growth, Turkey is an attractive destination for tourism as well as migration from neighboring countries by young people seeking employment opportunities. These trends put the country at increased risk for HIV/AIDS and further fuel misconceptions about HIV/AIDS that contribute to stigma and, especially, acquisition routes and externalization of blame. It is common in Muslim countries for people to equate HIV/AID with immoral sexual behavior and drug abuse with an assumption that the condition cannot be contracted if people are "morally correct," thus uniformly shaping all attitudes toward HIV/AIDS. In such circumstances, the social and cultural stigma is so great that the fear and exclusion, coupled with lack of knowledge about the true nature of the virus, has led to little compassion for people living with HIV/AIDS, let alone efforts to include them in daily activities or to respect their basic human rights. Global trends in stigma and HIV/AIDS are not of course unique to Turkey; nor are they unique to Muslim countries. Knowledge of HIV/AIDS is often equated with death as well as immorality; those who are living with HIV/AIDS are feared and blamed for spreading the virus. Already marginalized, many such groups are further stigmatized with the label of *high-risk group* without the requisite development of programs to address their problems. The media's role in representing HIV/AIDS as a disease of female sex workers and intravenous drug abusers continues to contribute to this negative picture. The corollary is that groups such as married couples and women may not be at risk, or are virtuous, thus ignoring changing trends in lifestyle and sexual behavior. Such poor social calibration resulting from the absence versus the presence of stigma is perhaps one of the biggest obstacles in the path to prevention. Cultural, educational, and religious institutions need to enter into a healthy dialogue with governmental and civic organizations to combat HIV/AIDS. This means that they need to be not only sufficiently informed, but have adequate sensitivity on the subject. The fight against HIV/AIDS needs to begin prior to an administration of an HIV test. Furthermore, HIV testing needs to be conducted with voluntary consent followed by voluntary counseling, after care and access to therapeutic options. The privacy of individuals with HIV infection should be protected; school nurses, principals, teachers, and personnel in workplace settings who have knowledge of a person's HIV status need to be absolutely required to keep the information confidential. While Turkey offers legal support for these mandates, policies and practices have not always aligned.

Conclusions

The involvement of young people as HIV/AIDS peer educators has the potential to help students become more knowledgeable about prevention, thus facilitating positive behavior change. The strength of peer education is its ability to prepare young people to effectively contribute to HIV/AIDS awareness in their social circle and school communities. Supervised training of adolescents to develop and deliver HIV/AIDS prevention messages to other youth is also a viable and effective means of increasing peer leaders' confidence in participating meaningfully in community health-prevention efforts.

Providing educational interventions by using peer educators or lectures is a viable means of HIV/AIDS education for positively impacting attitudes toward people with HIV/AIDS that may effect behavior change. Peer-education prevention programs demand a great deal of time commitment on the part of motivated young people. Peer educators must buy into HIV/AIDS prevention and apply these principles despite the social pressures and other barriers they may face. Yet, involvement of young people as HIV/AIDS peer educators, if sustained over time, has the potential for important social policy implications. Peer education can be a service delivery model among university counseling centers. Student personnel services can be strengthened by using peer-education service delivery modeled on HIV/AIDS prevention. It is also worth examining peer education as a service delivery model for its preventive and protective effects in terms of the mental health and physiological hygiene of youth. Youth-to-youth interventions have the potential for social policy-making implications. The role of young people as agents of change cannot be underestimated. For countries such as Turkey, where the HIV/AIDS epidemic is still at a dangerous yet formative stage, and where the population is youthful, both the peer-education and educational-lecture models can play an important preventive function and therefore need to be expanded.

There is an urgent need for developing and implementing policy and programs that provide HIV/AIDS education and awareness, prohibit stigmatization, and advocate compassion in schools. Like most religions, Islam condemns homosexuality, drug use, and sex outside marriage. Though the most important means of protection is obviously abstinence from sex and for marriage partners to remain faithful to each other, nevertheless, Turkish society must recognize that in many instances there is a gap between religious teaching and practice; risky behaviors that may not be allowed by Islam are indeed practiced. The main challenge is how to bridge this gap. This is a lesson not only in terms of efforts to prevent HIV/AIDS, but also in terms of sustaining a healthy framework for tolerance across global societies.

In this chapter we have underscored the notion of preventive education as a humanitarian response to HIV/AIDS. While peer-to-peer interventions certainly constitute one of the functional ways of using education to respond to a humanitarian need, information about staying healthy and reducing stigma can also mean ensuring inclusive education for children with stigmatized conditions. For education to be truly humanitarian, it must respond to the needs of the local situation. It often also needs to be guided by policies that might not be popular among, or accepted by, people holding contemporary values or alternatively those following traditional customs. In the case of Turkey, ensuring that children with HIV infection are allowed safe and inclusive education requires the additional education of the wider community about the rights and needs of people living with HIV/AID, as well as how the virus is transmitted. After all, in many developed countries, HIV/AIDS is no longer equated with death and how a good health prognosis can be achieved ought to be part and parcel of the educational process and a factor leading to tolerance. In order for stigma to decrease, more young Turks must feel sufficiently confident to be tested for STIs, receive appropriate treatment, and live long enough to dispel the myth that only the immoral become infected. Such examples would open more young minds to taking HIV/AIDS education seriously when it is provided.

References

Aggleton, P., and I. Warwick (2002). "Education and HIV/AIDS prevention among young people." *AIDS Education and Prevention* 14: 263–7.

AIDS Savaşım Derneği (AIDS Fight Society) (2002). Dünya AIDS Günü Basın Bülteni, 1 Aralık. [World AIDS Day press release, December 1].

Akyuz, E. (2000). "Ulusal ve Uluslararası Hukukta Çocuğun Haklarının ve Güvenliğinin Korunması" ["Rights of children and protection of security in national and international law"]. Ankara:.

Aras, S., S. Semin, T. Guncay, E. Orcin, and S. Ozan (2007). "Sexual attitudes and risk-taking behaviors of high-school students in Turkey." *Journal of School Health* 77 (7): 359–66.

Ay, P., and S. Karabey (2006). "Is there a 'hidden HIV/AIDS epidemic' in Turkey?: the gap between the numbers and the facts." *Marmara Medical Journal* 19 (2): 90–7.

Ayrancı, U. (2005). "AIDS knowledge and attitudes in a Turkish population: an epidemiological study." *BMC Public Health* 5, p. 95.

Babadoğan, C. (2002). *Akran eğitimi: Sosyal bilimler alanında eğitim gören üniversite gençliğinde HIV/ AIDS in önlenmesi [Peer education: Prevention of HIV/AIDS Among University Students Who Are Studying Social Sciences]*. Ankara, Turkey: Ankara University.

Backett–Milburn, K., and S. Wilson (2000). "Understanding peer education: insights from a process evaluation." *Health Education Research* 15 (1): 85–96.

Campbell C., and C. MacPhail (2002). "Peer education, gender and the development of critical consciousness: participatory HIV prevention by South African youth." *Social Science and Medicine* 55 (2): 331–45.

Campbell C., and Z. Mzaidume (2001). "Grassroots participation, peer education, and HIV prevention by sex workers in South Africa." *American Journal of Public Health* 91 (12): 1978–86.

Çelikbaş, A., O. Ergonul, N. Baykam, S. Eren, H. Esener, M. Eroglu, and B. Dokuzoguz (2008). "Epidemiologic and clinical characteristics of HIV/AIDS patients in Turkey, where the prevalence is the lowest in the region." *Journal of International Association of Physicians AIDS Care* 7 (1): 42–5.

Cok, F., L. A. Gray, and H. Ersever (2001). "Turkish university students' sexual behavior, knowledge, attitudes and perceptions of risk related to HIV/AIDS". *Culture, Health & Sexuality* 3: 81–99.

Duyan, V., and G. Yildirim (2003). "A brief picture of HIV/AIDS in Turkey." *AIDS Patient and Care and STDs* 17 (8): 373–5.

Ergene T., F. Cok. A. Tumer, and S. Unal (2005). "A controlled study of preventive effects of peer education and single-session lectures on HIV/AIDS knowledge and attitudes among university students in Turkey." *AIDS Education and Prevention : Official Publication of the International Society for AIDS Education* 17 (3): 268–78.

Eylen, B. (1996). "Öğrencilerin AIDS hakkındaki bilgi, tutum ve davranışları" ["Knowledge, attitudes and behaviors of students regarding AIDS"]. Paper presented at the Fourth Counseling and Guidance Congress, Çukurova University, Adana, Turkey.

Gökengin, D. (2002). "İlk ve ortaöğretimde HIV/AIDS ve diğer cinsel yolla bulaşan hastalıklardan korunma eğitimi." *HIV/AIDS* 5: 162–8.

Kontaş, M. (2003). "HIV/AIDS in Turkey." Paper presented at Sixth Turkish AIDS Congress, Istanbul, Turkey.

Medley, A., C. Kennedy, K. O'Reilly, and M. Sweat (2009). "Effectiveness of peer education interventions for HIV prevention in developing countries: a systematic review and meta-analysis." *AIDS Education and Prevention* 21 (3): 181–206.

Milburn, K. (1995). "A critical review of peer education with young people with special reference to sexual health." *Health Education Research* 10: 407–420.

Milliyet Newspaper (2003). www.milliyet.com.tr/2003/09/28/guncel/gun02.html [Accessed 13 June 2011].

Ministry of Health (2004). "Turkiye'de AIDS yayilimi" ["Prevalence of AIDS in Turkey"]. *Turkish Journal of AIDS* 20, p. 5.

— (2009). Ministry of Health Statistics Yearbook (2009). Ankara: İLTEK Publication.

Ornek Büken, N. (2006). "HIV/AIDS in Turkey and an HIV(+) child's right to education: Turkey's example." *Turk HIV/AIDS Dergisi* 9 (2): 37–46.

Ozcebe H., L. Akin, and D. Aslan (2004). "A peer education example on HIV/AIDS at a high school in Ankara." *Turkish Journal of Pediatrics* 46 (1): 54–9.

Ozeruz, B. (1999). *Lise ve yuksek ogrenime devam eden ogrencilerin cinsellige iliskin bilgi duzeylerinin arastirilmasi [The Research on Knowledge about Sexuality among Students Attending High School and Higher Education]* Master's degree thesis. Istanbul, Turkey: Marmara University.

Radikal Newspaper (2010). www.radikal.com.tr/Radikal.aspx?aType=RadikalDetayV3&ArticleID=98 7311&Date=23.03.2010&CategoryID=77 [Accessed 13 June 2011].

Turhan, E., Y. Inandi, and T. Inandi (2006). "Risk perception, knowledge and social distance of Turkish high school students about HIV/AIDS." *Journal of Public Health* 28 (2): 137–8.

Turkish Statistical Institute (2008). *Population Census Report of Turkey.* Ankara, Turkey: Turkish Statistical Institute Press.

UNAIDS (2003). *The Joint United Nations Program on HIV/AIDS: Geographical Area: Country— Turkey.* Geneva: UNAIDS.

Zeren, S. G. (2005). "HIV/AIDS'e yönelik önleyici çalışmalarda oyunun kullanılması." ["The use of play in HIV/AIDS prevention studies"]. *Eğitimde Yeni Yönelimler II, Eğitimde Oyun Sempozyumu, Özel Tevfik Fikret Okulları, 14 Mayıs, Ankara.(* New Directions in Education II, Educational Games Symposium, Tevfik Fikret Private Schools, May 14, Ankara).

Zeren, S. G., and T. Ergene (2008). "What kind of preventive activities school counselors can do about HIV/AIDS." *Elementary Education Online* 7 (1): 28–40.

Conclusion 8
Nalini Asha Biggs

What is education as a humanitarian response to HIV/AIDS?

Attempting to cover the many relationships between HIV/AIDS and education within one book is a monumental and arguably impossible task. These chapters have provided a handful of perspectives, however, on these relationships with the intention that education as a humanitarian response in a world where HIV/AIDS has become pandemic requires both global and local perspectives. While international cooperation and support is vital, as discussed by Christopher Castle and Mark Richmond's chapter, many of the other authors have described the nuanced challenges faced at local levels. David Clarke describes how across the Caribbean policy makers and researchers have recognized the importance of "knowing your epidemic" in order to adapt international policies for a local more-humanitarian response. David Kovara reviews how politics and culture in one country can make this difficult or impossible in another. Policy makers and researchers worldwide have many different views on the purpose of education. This book argues that education should be humanitarian, taking into account local needs of not only children in school but anyone engaged in the educational activity, and in essence should simply be "appropriate."

What is in store for the future of research and policy on these topics? For those specifically researching HIV/AIDS as an epidemic, there has been an influence from sociological perspectives and methods attempting to improve existing responses including educational interventions. "Evidence-informed" interventions now take into account lessons learned from qualitative research and small-scale studies focusing less on generalities and more on nuance. Researchers and policy makers from areas other than health sciences (such as social work, refugee studies and of course social science) are increasingly interested in the impact HIV/AIDS has on everything from politics to economics, from culture and the arts and even the physical environment. Mobile telecommunications and the Internet have significantly changed the way researchers define "education" and even "healthcare," with HIV tests becoming smaller, more mobile and less expensive everyday. While there is much bad news about HIV/AIDS, the potential of education is ever increasing.

Is HIV/AIDS a disability?

At the start of this book, I introduced a vignette about Deaf Kenyan women living in extreme poverty and at increased risk of becoming infected with HIV. Academics and advocates alike debate whether or not being Deaf is a "disability" or instead a linguistic difference. Much of the literature within disability studies is dedicated to debates over definitions and the theory of this pervasive idea. I myself as an academic and advocate have feet in both the fields of HIV/AIDS education and disability studies, and so I have wondered to what extent we can call HIV/AIDS a disability. Throughout this book authors make reference to the "disabling" aspects of AIDS, and indeed the greater body of this book discusses the importance of stigma in understanding this disease. At AIDS conferences and within the many tomes exploring HIV/AIDS there are scattered references to this linkage; this is not a new idea.

Currently most organizations (the World Health Organizations and United Nations agencies, for instance) define "disability" as being a little bit social and a little bit medical. "Disability," many now say, is a relationship between the individual and society where an impairment or disease (or simply a difference defined by society as undesirable) interacts with social stigma, exclusion and even oppression. There are entire libraries dedicated to better understanding and intense debate over what "is" and "is not" a disability. How does HIV/AIDS fit into this? How does education as a humanitarian response relate to this?

In the Series Editor's Preface, Colin Brock references this topic in terms of special education, and the need for children with disabilities to receive appropriate (humanitarian) education. In Tuncay Ergene and Kerim Munir's chapter, significant discussion is dedicated to the special needs of children living with HIV in formal schooling, and the protections that definition of "disability" in this case can bring.

If education as a "humanitarian response" means thinking about the *entire human* and shaping education *appropriate* to their needs, then for people with disabilities education must respond to both the individual impairment (or difference) *as well as* the social stigma and oppression they face. This book has repeatedly argued that while explicit HIV/AIDS prevention education is vital in reducing new infections, education can also help change the wider social structures that allow for this disease to be a pandemic in the first place. These authors have argued implicitly that education humanitarian response to HIV/AIDS takes into account *both* the medical realities of HIV and AIDS *as well as* the social stigmas causing and resulting from it. Are we in fact already talking about disability?

There is significant discomfort and resistance by many in using this label or identity, and indeed some disability activists can be equally dismayed by the idea of including HIV/AIDS into their circle of "real" disabilities. HIV/AIDS advocates and researchers alike have attempted to move away from people living with HIV being called "victims" of a "tragedy" or even "patients" seeing as they are not in a constant state of interaction with a medical professional. A life with HIV does not have to result in AIDS or an AIDS-related death. As more people are educated about the facts of this virus, stigma is decreasing and most are now aware that only an exchange of blood or semen is likely to infect, rather than hugs or sharing space as once were common myths. More and more people are realizing that much of the negative aspects of having HIV come from social stigma, persecution and lack of human rights. Similarly disability-focused international organizations and academics have moved away from the "victim" and "tragedy" discourses of disability as well. Yet colloquially the term "disability" still conjures up the kinds of images and ideas that HIV/AIDS activists are trying to move away from. Neither a person living with HIV nor someone who is, for instance, blind, wants to be thought of as "broken," "useless" or "infectious," yet they both often are.

Ironically, the ideals and goals of HIV/AIDS activists are the same as for disability activists: attempting to remove as much stigma as possible, increasing human rights while having access to the kinds of treatment and healthcare that can make the most out of people's lives. The struggles are almost parallel.

The stigmas that each group face also in many ways keep their political and social struggles apart for fear of "contamination" from either side (though the idea that "disability" is a homogenous group is as inaccurate as saying the same for PLWH). The resistance itself from either "side" warrants discussion. This is the final argument presented in this book: if we are to promote education as a humanitarian response to HIV/AIDS, we need to have a healthy debate over the usefulness of the term "disability" in this context.

Many do indeed discuss HIV/AIDS in terms of being a legally defined "disability" in order to protect employees from discrimination or patients attempting to secure or maintain healthcare. While "disability" is commonly viewed as an undesirable or even tragic condition defined by stigma, it can also be a protective label or identity ensuring rights or social sensitivity (see Gagnon and Stewart, 2008 for a detailed examination of one legal case where "disability" can be a positive, protective identity). While the identity or label of "disabled" might not be appropriate for someone who has HIV at all times (most people with disabilities argue the same for themselves), it can be useful for ensuring rights and even *lessening* stigma in some cases. Just as individuals are no longer "AIDS-patients" or "victims" but instead people living *with* HIV as one of *many* facets of their identity and experience, some of those experiences can be described as "disabling," in more ways than just physical or mental difficulties. The label and identity of "disabled" can stretch to encompass the stigma and oppression PLWH face from families, communities, employers and even their own governments.

I am not arguing that HIV/AIDS is in fact a "disability." Instead I am arguing that it is *useful* in the context of education as a humanitarian response to consider this perspective, often called the *social model* or a *social theory* of disability, in order to argue this cause. Including this perspective can strengthen the rationale for educational responses that seek to change more than individual behaviors. This perspective of disability reminds people to pay equal attention to society as a cause for the negative experiences faced by PLWH. It shifts focus away from education solely as a "vaccine" or "cure" (in the prevention sense) of a medical problem, and instead a tool for changing wider social issues that can negate or mitigate the need for more rigorous research on structural approaches.

Opening an explicit debate over the usefulness of discussing HIV/AIDS as a disability in some ways also helps disability advocates and researchers. We have long struggled over the significant lack of numbers justifying the need for funding and support for the rights (including most prominently for appropriate education) of people with disabilities in developing countries. Here there is an opportunity to widen the conversation. Much research has been dedicated to the vulnerabilities and challenges that orphans and children of people who have HIV/AIDS face. The same can be said about the children of parents with other significant disabilities: they are less likely to get an education, adequate nutrition and more likely to face abuse, neglect, and social stigma. Like HIV/AIDS, many disabilities are preventable, and a result of social inequalities that can be addressed by more general improvements in healthcare, education and human rights. Could these seemingly separate issues be strengthened by combining forces?

Concluding remarks

This book intends not to supply answers about "what works" necessarily, though many authors here have discussed positive outcomes from educational programs and successes in the response to HIV/AIDS. Instead it provides examples of different contexts, large and small, that education has responded to, at best in humanitarian ways. It also shows examples of when this has failed to occur, exploring the reasons for these failures and hopefully informing the reader on how future researchers, policy makers and practitioners can avoid these pitfalls. Finally, this book attempts to challenge the reader's preconceptions about the definition of "education," "humanitarian" and even finally "disability." These definitions will inevitably change as the world changes and, as this series argues, so will the overall meaning of "education as a humanitarian response."

Reference list

Gagnon, M. and M. Stuart. (2008). "Manufacturing disability: HIV, women and the construction of difference." *Nursing Philosophy* 10: 42–52.

Gupta, G. R., J. A. Ogden, J. O. Parkhurst, P. Aggleton, and A. Mahal. (2008). "Structural approaches to HIV prevention." *The Lancet* 372: 764–75.

Thomas, C. (2004) "How is disability understood? An examination of sociological approaches." *Disability & Society* 19 (6): 569–83.

Index